Falls in the Elderly

Joanna H. Downton
Consultant Geriatrician,
St Thomas' Hospital, Stockport

Edward Arnold

A division of Hodder & Stoughton

LONDON   MELBOURNE   AUCKLAND

© 1993 Joanna H. Downton

First published in Great Britain 1993

British Library Cataloguing in Publication Data

Downton, J. H.
  Falls in the Elderly
  I. Title
  618.97

  ISBN 0–340–54848–7

Whilst the advice and information in this book is believed to be true and accurate at the date of going to press, neither the author nor the publisher can accept any legal responsibility or liability for any errors or omissions that may be made. In particular (but without limiting the generality of the preceding disclaimer) every effort has been made to check drug dosages; however, it is still possible that errors have been missed. Furthermore, dosage schedules are constantly being revised and new side effects recognised. For these reasons the reader is strongly urged to consult the drug companies' printed instructions before administering any of the drugs recommended in this book.

Typeset in 10/12pt Times by Wearset, Boldon, Tyne and Wear. Printed and bound in Great Britain for Edward Arnold, a division of Hodder & Stoughton Limited, Mill Road, Dunton Green, Sevenoaks, Kent TN13 2YA by Biddles Ltd., Guildford and King's Lynn

Preface

Many doctors recognise 'heart-sink' patients – those with vague, persistent and intractable problems. For people providing medical and social care for the elderly, falls and dizziness are frequently 'heart-sink' complaints. Symptoms may be vague or indefinable, the underlying problems are frequently multifactorial, and it is often thought that such disorders are an inevitable result of ageing. What I hope to achieve with this book is to demonstrate that it is possible in most cases to unravel the complaints sufficiently to understand what is happening, and to intervene to ameliorate the situation. Even if further falls cannot be prevented, it is rare that there is 'nothing to be done' to improve the situation of the faller. The negative and dismissive attitude which such complaints often engender is as unnecessary for falls as it is for the other 'Geriatric Giants'.

A number of people have helped me with this book. I would like to thank Wendy Stewart and Peggy Brookes for helpful comments on Chapter 8, and the staff of the Physiotherapy Department and the Day Hospital at St Thomas' Hospital, Stockport and the Department of Medical Illustration, Withington Hospital for assistance with the photographs. Ray Tallis provided much useful advice and encouragement, for which I am very grateful. Most of all I would like to thank Martin for being exceptionally patient.

J. Downton
1992

Contents

Chapter 1 _____

Facts and uncertainties – the epidemiology of falls

A previously healthy 82 year-old woman fell at home whilst walking across the sitting room. She was unable to get up and looked pale and unwell, so her husband called an ambulance. At the Accident and Emergency Department an electrocardiogram (ECG) was performed which showed an acute anterior myocardial infarction.

A 77 year-old woman was walking her dog when he attempted to chase a cat. She was pulled off balance and fell, fracturing her wrist.

A frail 93 year-old man lived independently at home despite poor vision, severe osteoarthritis and mild Parkinson's disease. He had recurrent falls, which on assessment were felt to be due to a combination of poor balance (visual impairment and Parkinson's disease), unstable knee joints (osteoarthritis), postural hypotension (medication for Parkinson's disease) and iron-deficiency anaemia (caused by non-steroidal anti-inflammatory drug treatment).

A 75 year-old man with a history of ischaemic heart disease described recurrent falls associated with transient loss of consciousness. A 24-hour ECG recording demonstrated recurrent episodes of ventricular tachycardia. His symptoms were abolished by treatment with an anti-arrhythmic drug.

Old people fall. Their instability and tendency to fall is widely recognised and, rightly or wrongly, accepted as a fact of ageing. The cases described above demonstrate, however, that there are many potential causes. As with other non-specific symptoms with which health problems in the elderly may present, an assumption that the problem is purely related to ageing ('It's just your age, dear') sometimes means that assessment of treatable problems is delayed, and avoidable disability and dependence may result. There are significant medical, economic and social consequences that follow from this tendency of old people to fall, and with the projected increase in the elderly, particularly the very elderly, these are likely to become increasingly important.

To plan health and social care appropriately the scale of the problem must be assessed. This means that there are a number of questions that need to be answered. First, and most importantly, who falls and why; that is, are there particular groups of elderly at high risk of falling, either by reason of some quirk of their physiology or because of particular disease processes? Secondly, how do falls occur? This implies looking at the mechanisms that maintain balance most of the time, and at the age- and disease-related changes that take place in the elderly which may compromise balance. Thirdly, when and where do falls occur? Particular environmental factors that are risky for the elderly need to be identified. In other words, we need to know about the epidemiology of falls – not a simple matter.

There are a number of problems which beset those wishing to study the epidemiology of falls. Falls are common, but unpredictable. 'Falling' covers a wide range of problems, from apparently minor trips and slips to events causing serious and sometimes life-threatening injury. There is a continuum from trips and stumbles, when balance is regained, through near falls to completed falls. The fact that falls occur at all stages of life means that they seem to be unremarkable, everyday events, not worthy of being reported. There is also an embarrassment factor which dissuades people from bringing them to the attention of family, carers or health workers. The association with loss of control (and the joking comments about alcohol – 'you should take more water with it!'), and the fear that falling may lead to enforced loss of independence sometimes results in shame and unwillingness to admit to falls. There is a paradox of falls being mundanely understandable and common, yet inexplicable. All of these factors mean that many falls are not reported and may in fact not be remembered by the faller.

The next problem is that falls seem to be commonest in groups that are not typical of all old people, such as those living in institutional care, which means that information about features and causes of falls in those groups cannot necessarily be extrapolated or generalised to all elderly people. It is likely that there are situations (and groups of elderly) in which the risk of falling is high for physiological or pathological reasons and other groups and situations in which risk of falling is low. Any group of elderly will be a mix of people with different intrinsic risks of falling, in different environments, with different lifestyles putting them at high, low or intermediate risk. It is therefore important to study a sample that is randomly selected, to include a typical cross-section of the population being considered, and also to characterise the sample so that comparisons with other groups (and other studies) can be made. Many studies have used subject groups which are not randomly selected, often with insufficient information available to identify the sort of old people studied. For example, there is quite a lot of information available about the frequency and causes of falls amongst those in hospital or institutional care, but criteria for admission to these facilities vary from country to country, and even from area to area within a country. Findings from these studies cannot, therefore, be extrapolated to elderly people in general.

Information about the frequency of falls can be obtained by studying those who suffer injury from falls, those who may or may not be injured but who report their falls, or by retrospectively or prospectively studying various populations of elderly people. It will be clear that these groups are not equivalent. Studies looking at the prevalence of falling have come up with estimates of frequency of falls which have varied from 23 per cent to 59 per cent of old people in hospital or institutional care and from 28 per cent to 60 per cent of old people at home (Downton, 1987). These discrepancies may result from genuine large differences in prevalence of falling between and within populations, but are more likely to indicate methodological problems arising from the difficulties discussed above.

Those who are known to have fallen, usually because they have presented to medical attention (either to hospital or to their general practitioner (GP) or other primary care worker), probably make up less than half of all fallers, and the proportion may be much less than that. Estimates of the rate of falls from data collected for the Home Accident Surveillance System (HASS), which gathers information about those attending hospital Accident and Emergency Departments in England and Wales following accidents at home, suggest that approximately 20 per 1000 of the population aged 60+ are affected (Consumer Safety Unit, 1988), whereas the estimates of frequency of falls amongst community elderly are more than tenfold greater than this.

Old people presenting with a specific injury are in some ways a much easier group to study because most will present to hospital (or to other sources of medical aid) for treatment. However, because only a small proportion of falls result in injuries requiring medical treatment, the findings from studies of those with injuries will not necessarily apply to all fallers.

Most of the studies of falls in old people in hospital are difficult to interpret because the study population is often not defined, for example in classifications such as '100 ambulant patients'. The age and sex characteristics of the population may not be stated, and when studies involve American Veterans Administration hospitals, where patients are predominantly men and often younger than 65 years, or where hospital populations of all ages are considered, it can be particularly difficult to know whether results can be generalised. Studies of old people in residential care are similarly difficult to interpret and compare. The populations considered are obviously selected but with characteristics that are likely to vary because of different systems of care for old people.

A large majority of old people in the United Kingdom (approximately 95 per cent) are living in the community in their own homes rather than in residential care. Other Western countries have similar figures. Despite the fact that those old people who are in hospital or residential care are almost certainly frailer and probably more liable to suffer from complications of falls (Wilkin et al., 1978) the fact that such a large proportion of the elderly is living at home suggests that the majority of falls and their complications will occur in this group. This is borne out by HASS data, which showed that in 1987 84.2 per cent of accidents to people over 60 occurred to those living in their own homes (Consumer Safety Unit, 1988) Old people at home could therefore be said to be the most important group in which to study the epidemiology of falls.

Selecting a study sample may not be straightforward. Ideally the whole of a population at risk should be studied, but the logistics of this kind of study are usually difficult. It is therefore more realistic and manageable to choose a proportion of the population for study, and this should be a randomly chosen section of the elderly population of an area. Conclusions drawn from such studies are more likely to be generally applicable, though socio-economic differences between areas may complicate interpretation of results and comparisons between studies.

Once an appropriate study population has been chosen, the next problem is deciding what constitutes a fall. Defining a fall can be difficult. Some studies look at accidents in general, and though a large proportion of accidents in the elderly are falls, this will include a variable proportion of non-fall events. Others exclude specific types of falls such as those involving loss of consciousness or acute medical illness, or unwitnessed falls. Sometimes only accidents requiring medical investigation and treatment are included, and in some cases only falls in or close to the home are considered. This is probably an artificial and unhelpful distinction, as a quarter to a half of falls reported occur out of doors, and the proportion of fallers having their falls outdoors may be higher in the 'healthy elderly' (Gabell et al., 1985).

In institutionalised subjects much of the available information comes from retrospective inspection of accident forms. Such forms are largely filled in for medico-legal reasons, and it is likely for example that a very high proportion of falls resulting in injury are reported, whereas falls without injury, particularly if unwitnessed, may be omitted. The forms will probably have been filled in by many different staff members, each likely to have differing criteria and thresholds for reporting incidents, with a resulting lack of standardisation.

Reliability of history is a general and probably unavoidable problem, especially with any retrospective study or study of community-living elderly. A retrospective study (other than one using accident forms) will depend on the subjects' memory of falls that have occurred. There is some evidence that subjects with cognitive impairment are more likely to fall, so those who are most at risk of falling may be least likely to remember their falls. More recently, various schemes for prospective ascertainment of falls have been devised, which mostly depend on investigators contacting subjects regularly to ask about falls. It is still possible that some falls will escape reporting, particularly in those with memory impairment. The factors discussed above, relating to embarrassment about falling, or fear of institutionalisation, also mean that falls may be consciously or subconsciously under-reported.

A study specifically looking at accuracy of retrospective recall of falls in the elderly found that 13 per cent of those with documented falls over a 12 month period failed to recall these falls at the end of that time. Surprisingly, recall was less accurate if the recall period was three or six months rather than 12, and there were only weak correlations between the number of falls that were documented and the number that were recalled during each of these periods (Cummings et al., 1988).

Epidemiology of falling

How common are falls?

Many of the early studies of the epidemiology of falls suffered from one or more of the methodological problems outlined above, but more recently there have been a number of much sounder studies, particularly amongst 'free-range', community-living elderly, so there is now much clearer information about how common falls are, and what factors are associated with an increased risk of falling in these populations. Studies of the frequency of falls in more or less randomly selected community populations have all produced similar annual prevalence rates: 28–35 per cent for subjects aged 65+ (Campbell et al., 1981; Prudham and Evans, 1981; Blake et al., 1988), 35 per cent for those aged 70+ (Campbell et al., 1989) and 32–42 per cent for those aged 75+ (Tinetti et al., 1988; Downton and Andrews, 1991). 'Healthy elderly' are less likely to fall (Gabell et al., 1985), but those who have already fallen are more likely to fall again. Of those who have fallen in the previous year, 60–70 per cent are likely to fall during the following 12 months (Nevitt et al., 1989).

It is more difficult to draw conclusions about the incidence or prevalence of falls in the elderly in institutional care, because populations are not necessarily comparable, and because some studies look at falls specifically while others look at 'accidents'. However, falls amongst these groups of elderly are very common and are almost certainly commoner than amongst the elderly in the community. It is likely that at least half of the elderly in institutional care will fall in the course of a year.

Studies of hospital fallers are particularly difficult to compare with one another because of the many different ways in which fall rates are expressed. Examples include accident rate per occupied bed per year, fall rate per 10 000 patient days, fall rate per 1000 bed occupation days, accident rate per 1000 patients admitted, accidents per bed day or per patient day and falls as a percentage of total discharges.

When and where do falls occur?

Between a quarter and a half of falls occur away from home. Of those falls in and around the home, most occur where people spend most time, as might be expected. Of falls around the home requiring attention at Accident Departments, two thirds occur in the house, and of these, almost three quarters happen in the kitchen, living/dining room or bedroom (Consumer Safety

Unit, 1988). Only a small proportion of falls occur on stairs, though such falls are more likely to result in significant injury. Most falls occur during the day (Downton and Andrews, 1991), which again is what would be expected since falls usually occur during movement or activity of some kind.

Falls occurring away from home are more likely to occur to healthy elderly, and the risk of injury is higher than for falls in and around the home (Speechley and Tinetti, 1991).

What factors are associated with falls?

Much work has been done and many studies published on the subject of the cause of falls. There are the same problems of subject selection, definitions, and reliability of history as with determining the frequency of falls. In addition there are further problems. Falls are almost always caused by combinations of intrinsic and extrinsic factors. A particular factor or factors may put someone at risk of falling, but will not guarantee that a fall will occur. Even someone at very high risk of falling will only fall intermittently, because of the interaction of intrinsic, environmental and situational factors. This may partially explain the confusing and contradictory findings of the many studies, from which one could demonstrate that almost any factor is and is not associated with falls. However, there are some factors which seem to be fairly consistently associated with an altered risk of falling.

Age and sex
Virtually all studies have shown increasing risk of falling with increasing age and most have shown women to be more likely to fall than men, though the reverse appears to be true in hospital (Berry et al., 1981), perhaps because men in hospital, particularly those in continuing care areas, tend to be especially frail and disabled (and often more so than women because they are more likely to have been supported at home in the earlier stages of their disability by a female relative). In some studies the very elderly have a lower incidence of falls, perhaps because of selective survival of a particularly fit cohort (Prudham and Evans, 1981; Woodhouse et al., 1983). Amongst those in institutional care, the 'young elderly' (those under 75) seem to be more prone to fall (Haga et al., 1986), possibly because those requiring institutional care at a 'young' age are almost always very physically and/or mentally frail.

Drugs
The evidence here is confused, partly because of the difficulty of separating the effects of drugs from the effects of the diseases for which they are prescribed. In general terms, a large proportion of old people take both prescribed and over-the-counter drugs, and because of changes in pharmaco-kinetics and pharmacodynamics with ageing are more liable to suffer side effects from drug therapy (Anonymous, 1988). In general, consumption of

any drug may be associated with an increase in the likelihood of falling (Prudham and Evans, 1981).

Theoretically, drugs likely to be implicated are those which may have an effect on postural stability either because of their central depressant effect (e.g. minor tranquillisers, sedatives, hypnotics), because they are liable to cause postural hypotension (e.g. antihypertensives), or both (e.g. tricyclic antidepressants, major tranquillisers). In each of these cases, there has been found to be an association between consumption of the drugs and either falling per se or fractures secondary to falls (MacDonald and MacDonald, 1977; Tinker, 1979; Wild et al., 1980; Davie et al., 1981; Campbell et al., 1981; Blake et al., 1988). However, there also seem to be risks with other drugs, for example non-steroidal anti-inflammatory drugs which can produce symptoms of dizziness in elderly people (Goodwin and Regan, 1982). There may be differences between specific drugs within groups, for instance long and short half-life hypnotics (Ray et al., 1987). Long half-life hypnotics are more likely to produce 'hang-over' sedation the following day, with potential effects on stability and alertness, and may accumulate with chronic use. Nitrazepam, which is still commonly taken as night sedation by elderly people in the UK, has a half-life even in healthy young people of 20 hours or more, and in the elderly the half-life may be up to 60 hours (Swift, 1983). Accumulation is therefore almost inevitable with regular use.

The evidence concerning diuretics is conflicting. There is some evidence that thiazides protect against fracture because they reduce loss of calcium from the body due to a hypocalciuric effect (Rashiq and Logan, 1986). However, those taking diuretics have a high incidence of symptoms of dizziness, fainting and blacking out (Hale et al., 1984). Associations have been reported between thiazide intake and femoral fracture (Muckle, 1976), injury following a fall (Whitlock et al., 1978), and falls themselves (Prudham and Evans, 1981).

Little is known about the relationship between alcohol consumption and falls, particularly in the elderly. Information about fatal home accidents in Sweden, based on death certification (Berfenstam et al., 1969) showed that alcohol was implicated in half of poisonings, a quarter of fire deaths, but only 5 per cent of fall deaths (though many elderly people dying as a result of falls were not included in the study, for reasons that were not stated). Blood alcohol levels above 50 mg/100 ml substantially increase the risk of falling in adults (Honkanen et al., 1983), and it therefore seems likely that alcohol increases the risk of falling. However, where the association has been considered, alcohol has been implicated in only small proportions of falls in the elderly (Waller, 1978; Turner et al., 1990). Under-reporting is likely.

There is, however, one group of elderly fallers where alcohol is clearly implicated – those with head injury (Pentland et al., 1986). Alcohol is a contributory factor in about a third of head-injured elderly overall, and alcohol-related head injuries are commoner in males than females. Over half of minor head injuries in elderly males requiring admission to hospital are alcohol-related, and there does not seem to be much difference between elderly and young male head injury victims as far as alcohol as a contributing factor is concerned.

Cognitive function

It is well recognised that cognitive impairment is common in old people who have suffered a fractured neck of femur, but as these measurements are made at variable times after the injury, some of this may be related to the injury itself, treatment of the injury (e.g. the effects of a general anaesthetic), or the illness which may have precipitated the fall. Fallers have in general been found to have a higher prevalence of cognitive impairment than non-fallers (Prudham and Evans, 1981; Campbell et al., 1981), and subjects with dementia are as much as three times more likely to fall than non-demented controls (Morris et al., 1987).

Postural control

Gait and balance have often been considered though frequently in a subjective way, for example in statements such as mobility being 'more impaired' in some groups of fallers (Campbell et al., 1981). Subjectively assessed gait has been noted to be abnormal in many studies, and studies using more objective measurements have found some associations between impaired gait and balance and risk of falling, though there is a substantial overlap between fallers and non-fallers. This will be considered in more detail in Chapter 4.

Dependency

Statistically significant associations between difficulty getting about indoors, difficulty getting in and out of bed and difficulty dressing, and whether falls had been reported in the past year have been found, though the differences were 'not striking in magnitude' (Prudham and Evans, 1981). The New Zealand community study reported reduced 'functional ability' in pattern fallers compared with non-fallers and occasional fallers, classifying functional disability as none, mild, marked or severe, though no information was given about how these categories were allocated (Campbell et al., 1981). Frail elderly with multiple health problems, who also often have recurrent falls, tend to have higher dependency levels than their fitter peers.

Other factors

Numerous other factors have been found to be associated with falls in individual studies and contradictory findings have been reported from diffe-rent studies. Many factors are implicated and it seems likely that combina-tions of factors are more important than single problems. Many of the factors are likely to be interdependent, for example age and cognitive function, confusion and dependency, and neurological disease and abnormal gait.

Although there are statistical associations between the various factors and falls it is still very difficult to disentangle the relative risk of any particular factor, and an association between a particular factor and falling does not prove causation. The causes of falls are considered further in Chapter 5.

Types of falls

There are probably two main types of falls – trip/slip and 'non-trip', though in practice distinguishing between the two can be difficult. In many studies, fallers have been subdivided into different groups, for example occasional fallers and pattern fallers, single falls and multiple falls, trips and non-trip falls, and few and many falls. There are problems in these classifications because they often rely on the subject's own description, even if the fall is witnessed, and old people frequently seem to be very vague about what happened. They often seem to rationalise: 'I must have tripped.' In addition there is often a subjective element to the classifications, and the multifactorial causation of falls also leads to difficulties.

In general three categories have been used; intrinsic, extrinsic and 'other'. The extrinsic group consists of trips, slips, and other environmentally caused falls, the 'other' group mainly of unknown or 'don't know' responses and the intrinsic group covers a wide range of problems (with variation depending on the particular study, and sometimes on the interests of the observer) including medical episodes, dizziness, 'loss of balance', drop attacks, blackouts, 'legs giving way' and various other categories.

In practical terms it may be possible to classify falls into trips/slips and non-trip falls though this may underestimate the number of falls due to simple trips. An alternative classification based on what the faller was doing at the time of the fall has been suggested (Isaacs, 1978), but this seems to be equally subjective (for example, 'a fall resulting from an encounter, during normal movement, with a hazard which could have been perceived and avoided'). A more rigorous classification system has been devised, using clear operational definitions, with good inter-rater reliability, and allowing grouping of falls in many ways for analysis (Lach et al., 1991). Falls can be classified on the basis of the subjects description of the fall and its circumstances into four main groups (extrinsic, intrinsic, non-bipedal, ie falls from bed or chair, and unclassified), with sub-classifications that allow the probable cause of the fall to be decided and contributing factors to be included. No information is yet available about how useful this classification is in the practical management of falls and fallers.

The rationale behind subdividing falls in some way is that falls occur at all ages if balance mechanisms are sufficiently stressed, but elderly people seem much more prone to falling in situations of relatively minor 'balance stress'. It seems possible that falls occurring in these circumstances have different causes from 'a genuine slip such as might happen to anyone' (Sheldon, 1948). However, the difficulties of ensuring an accurate account of the exact circumstances of the fall mean that differences between the types are blurred. It also seems likely that those who have multiple falls have different characteristics from those with a single fall, but it is only with the benefit of hindsight that such a distinction can be made – a single fall may be the first of many.

No studies have been reported in which subdivisions of types of fall have been used in the assessment or management of elderly fallers, but these subdivisions theoretically have some practical use in the management of fallers.

References

Anonymous (1988). Need we poison the elderly so often? (Editorial). *Lancet.* **2:** 20–22.

Berfenstam, R., Lagerberg, D. and Smedby, B. (1969). Victim characteristics in fatal home accidents. *Acta Socio-med Scand.* **1:** 145–164.

Berry, G., Fisher, R.H. and Lang, S. (1981). Detrimental incidents, including falls, in an elderly institutional population. *J Am Geriatr Soc.* **29:** 322–324.

Blake, A.J., Morgan, K., Bendall, M.J., Dallosso, H., Ebrahim, S.B.J., Arie, T.H.D., Fentem, P.H. and Bassey, E.J. (1988). Falls by elderly people at home: prevalence and associated factors. *Age Ageing.* **17:** 365–372.

Campbell, A.J., Borrie, M.J. and Spears, G.F. (1989). Risk factors for falls in a community-based prospective study of people 70 years and older. *J Gerontol.* **44:** M112–117.

Campbell, A.J., Reinken, J., Allan, B.C. and Martinez, G.S. (1981). Falls in old age: a study of frequency and related clinical factors. *Age Ageing.* **10:** 264–270.

Consumer Safety Unit (1988). *Home and Leisure Accident Research.*

Cummings, S.R., Nevitt, M.C. and Kidd, S. (1988). Forgetting falls. The limited accuracy of recall of falls in the elderly. *J Am Geriatr Soc.* **36:** 613–616.

Davie, J.W., Blumenthal, M.D. and Robinson-Hawkins, S. (1981). A model of risk of falling for psychogeriatric patients. *Arch Gen Psych.* **38:** 463–467.

Downton, J. (1987). The problems of epidemiological studies of falls. *Clin Rehab.* **1:** 243–246.

Downton, J.H. and Andrews, K. (1991). Prevalence, characteristics and factors associated with falls among the elderly living at home. *Aging.* **3:** 219–228.

Gabell, A., Simons, M.A. and Nayak, U.S.L. (1985). Falls in the healthy elderly: predisposing causes. *Ergonomics.* **28:** 965–975.

Goodwin, J.S. and Regan, M. (1982). Cognitive dysfunction associated with naproxen and ibuprofen in the elderly. *Arthr Rheum.* **25:** 1013–1014.

Haga, H., Shibata, H., Shichita, K., Matsuzaki, T. and Hatano, S. (1986). Falls in the institutionalised elderly in Japan. *Arch Gerontol Geriatr.* **5:** 1–9.

Hale, W.E., Stewart, R.B. and Marks, R.G. (1984). Central nervous system symptoms of elderly subjects using antihypertensive drugs. *J Am Geriatr Soc.* **32:** 5–10.

Honkanen, R., Ertama, L., Kuosmanen, P., Linnoila, M., Alha, A. and Visuri, T. (1983). The role of alcohol in accidental falls. *J Stud Alcohol.* **44:** 231–254.

Isaacs, B. (1978). Are falls a manifestation of brain failure? *Age Ageing.* **7 (Suppl):** 97–105.

Lach, H.W., Reed, A.T., Arfken, C.L., Miller, J.P., Paige, G.D., Birge, S.J. and Peck, W.A. (1991). Falls in the elderly: reliability of a classification system. *J Am Geriatrics Soc.* **39:** 197–202.

MacDonald, J.B. and MacDonald, E.T. (1977). Nocturnal femoral fracture and continuing widespread use of barbiturate hypnotics. *Br Med J*. **2**: 483–485.

Morris, J.C., Rubin, E.H., Morris, E.J., Mandel, S.A. (1987). Senile dementia of the Alzheimer's type: an important risk factor for serious falls. *J Gerontol*. **42**: 412–417.

Muckle, D.S. (1976). Iatrogenic factors in femoral neck fractures. *Injury*. **8**: 98–101.

Nevitt, M.C., Cummings, S.R., Kidd, S. and Black, D. (1989). Risk factors for recurrent non-syncopal falls. A prospective study. *JAMA*. **261**: 2663–2668.

Pentland, B., Jones, P.A., Roy, C.W. and Miller, J.D. (1986). Head injury in the elderly. *Age Ageing*. **15**: 193–202.

Prudham, D., Evans, J.G. (1981). Factors associated with falls in the elderly: a community study. *Age Ageing*. **10**: 141–146.

Rashiq, S. and Logan, R.F.A. (1986). Role of drugs in fractures of the femoral neck. *Br Med J*. **292**: 861–863.

Ray, W.A., Griffin, M.R., Shaffner, W., Baugh, D.K. and Melton, L.J. (1987). Psychotropic drug use and the risk of hip fracture. *N Engl J Med*. **316**: 363–369.

Sheldon, J.H. (1948). *The Social Medicine of Old Age. Report of an inquiry in Wolverhampton*. London, Oxford University Press.

Speechley, M. and Tinetti, M. (1991). Falls and injuries in frail and vigorous community elderly persons. *J Am Geriatr Soc*. **39**: 46–52.

Swift, C.G. (1983). Hypnotic drugs. In *Recent Advances in Geriatric Medicine*. Isaacs, B. (ed.). Edinburgh: Churchill Livingstone, pp. 123–146.

Tinetti, M.E., Speechley, M. and Ginter, S.F. (1988). Risk factors for falls among elderly persons living in the community. *N Engl J Med*. **319**: 1701–1707.

Tinker, G.M. (1979). Accidents in a geriatric department. *Age Ageing*. **8**: 196–198.

Turner, G.F., Wilson, P., Ward, G., James, S. and Legg, E.F. (1990). What proportion of falls in elderly people who present to hospital are related to alcohol drinking? *Care of the Elderly*. **2**: 413–414.

Waller, J.A. (1978). Falls among the elderly – human and environmental factors. *Accid Anal Prev*. **10**: 21–33.

Whitlock, F.A., Boyce, L. and Siskind, V. (1978). Accidents in old age. *Aus Fam Phys*. **7**: 389–399.

Wild, D., Nayak, U.S.L. and Isaacs, B. (1980). Characteristics of old people who fell at home. *J Clin Exp Gerontol*. **2**: 271–278.

Wilkin, D., Mashiah, T. and Jolley, D.J. (1978). Changes in behavioural characteristics of elderly populations of local authority homes and long-stay hospital wards 1976–7. *Br Med J*. **2**: 1274–1276.

Woodhouse, P.R., Briggs, R.S. and Ward, D. (1983). Falls and disability in old peoples homes. *J Clin Exp Gerontol*. **5**: 309–321.

Chapter 2 _____

The consequences of falling for the elderly and society

Introduction

The consequences of falls may be serious at any age, but to the elderly they have significance beyond that in younger people. These consequences can be direct physical effects such as injury or death, or less direct effects of increased dependency and impaired self-care, leading to demands on carers or to residential or nursing home placement. The psychological effects can be profound, even in the absence of significant physical injury. There are also important economic implications for society, because of the resulting use of health care, or need for social care.

Complications of falls

Death due to falls

Death following a fall may result directly from injuries sustained by falling, or may follow complications of the fall or the injury, such as pneumonia or hypothermia. There is a significant operative and postoperative mortality resulting from surgical treatment of fractured neck of femur and other injuries. The fall may be a non-specific marker of an illness which itself may lead to death.

Most deaths due to falls occur in the elderly. About three quarters of such deaths are in those over 65 years of age (Eddy, 1973), and approximately 0.15 per cent per year of those over 65 die from accidental falls (Lucht, 1971). Information about fatal accidents at home in England and Wales is available from the Home Accident Death Database (Consumer Safety Unit, 1988), and in 1985 falls accounted for 62 per cent of all fatal home accidents and 78 per cent of fatal home accidents in those aged 65+. Nearly 90 per cent of deaths due to falls at home were in those over 65.

In the USA, trauma is the fifth largest cause of death in the over 65s, and two-thirds of these injuries are caused by falls (Oreskovich et al., 1984). In the UK, falls account for 63 per cent and 82 per cent of all fatal non-transport accidents in the 65–74 and 75+ age groups respectively (Askham et al., 1990). Because of bone fragility and failure of protective reflexes, the elderly are more likely to injure themselves if they fall, and because of age- and disease-related impairment of physiological responses and homeostatic reserve are five times more likely to die from injuries of equivalent severity than the young. Available figures may underestimate the scale of the problem, since late deaths are not always correctly certified.

Death certification is well known to be inaccurate, and miscertification is probably commoner for the elderly than the young. In addition, if an old person dies from a complication of a fall, such as pneumonia or hypothermia, particularly if the death occurs some time after the fall, the fall may not appear on the certificate. People dying from falls are less likely to have an autopsy than those dying from other accidents (Berfenstam et al., 1969), and in contrast to younger people dying following an accident, the elderly accident victim is much less likely to have the accident mentioned on the death certificate (Fife and Rappaport, 1987). Thus death rates from injuries in the elderly are likely to be substantially more than those suggested by death certificate data.

Fatal accidental falls in the home are almost exclusively a problem of the elderly. They affect less than 10 per 100 000 under the age of 65, but the incidence then rises exponentially (Fig. 2.1).

Marker for likelihood of death

Falls seem to be a marker of increasing frailty and risk of dying. Anecdotal reports have described a fall as a herald of impending deterioration, and clustering of falls prior to death has been reported in residents of a home for the elderly, in whom those with many falls had a particularly high death rate (Gryfe et al., 1977).

The mortality rate of old people who have fallen seems to be greater than that of a control non-falling population, particularly for those in hospital and for the generally frail (Naylor and Rosin, 1970; Wild et al., 1981). Being unable to get up from the floor and consequently suffering a 'long lie' signals a particularly high risk of death. One study found that half of those who remained on the floor for an hour or more died within the next six months (Wild et al., 1981).

A prospective study of falls in a representative community population found that male but not female fallers had a significantly greater risk of dying (over a period of follow-up of 40 to 46 months) than non-fallers (Campbell et al., 1990). Falls were one of several factors found to be significant predictors of mortality in a follow-up study of a community population, and were felt to demonstrate underlying frailty or illness rather than being a direct cause of death (Campbell et al., 1985). In elderly subjects attending accident depart-

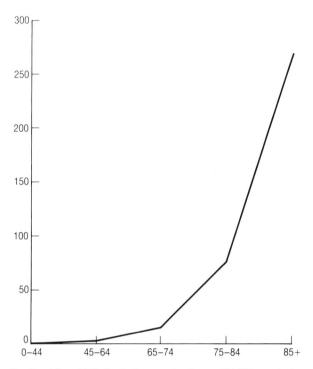

Fig. 2.1   Fatal accidental falls in the home – deaths per 100 000 population per year
data from Berfenstam et al., 1969

ments following a fall at home, mortality rate was double that expected over
the following 12 months, and those in whom a health factor rather than an
environmental factor was identified as the cause of the fall were particularly
likely to die during the year after their fall (Morfitt, 1983).

Injuries due to falls

Most serious injuries and the majority of fractures in the elderly are caused by
falling (Oreskovich et al., 1984; Melton and Riggs, 1987), and injuries, largely
due to falls, are common reasons for elderly people to attend Accident and
Emergency Departments (Dove and Dave, 1986). Falls account for about 60
per cent of all injuries in the elderly and this is a greater proportion than in
other age groups (Fig. 2.2). Fractures are discussed in more detail in Chapter
3. Injuries other than fractures have not been studied in as much detail, and
reports of injuries due to falls in the elderly in general do not separate
fractures from other injuries.

Injury rates overall (i.e. total injuries from all causes) are lower in the
elderly than the young, but the elderly have a higher case fatality and
disability rate following injury (Hogue, 1982). The long term consequences of
a fall-related injury can be devastating, particularly for those with severe

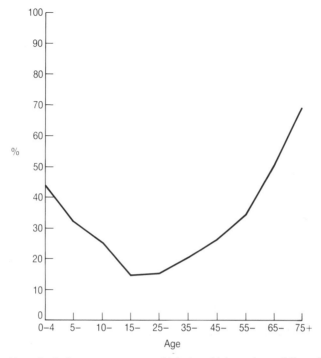

Fig. 2.2   Accidents in the home – percentage of injuries which are due to falls at different ages data from Home and Leisure Accident Research, Home Accident Surveilance System (HASS), 1987

injury. An American study of serious injuries in over-70 year olds (of which about three-quarters were caused by falls) found that although 85 per cent survived, very few regained sufficient independence to live alone, and the majority ended up in long-term nursing care (Oreskovich et al., 1984), though it is not clear how far this was due to inadequate community support systems.

In general, injury of some sort seems to occur in about half of those who fall (Downton and Andrews, 1991), but less than 10 per cent of fallers suffer fractures (Campbell et al., 1990). 'Healthy' or 'vigorous' elderly seem at higher risk of injury despite a lower risk of falls (Gabell et al., 1985; Speechley and Tinetti, 1991).

Estimates of population incidence of injuries from falls vary from country to country, perhaps reflecting different systems of medical care and differential access to health services. In a poor black urban community in the USA, 26 per 1000 of the population aged 65+ were treated at an Emergency Department for injuries following falls. Fall injuries made up almost half of all injuries in this age group, and unlike other injuries, increased in incidence with increasing age (Grisso et al., 1990). A Swedish study of injuries following falls at home found an incidence of 14 per 1000 aged 60+ (Lucht, 1971). Again incidence increased with age.

Approximately half of elderly attenders of Accident and Emergency

Departments in the UK have suffered trauma (Dove and Dave, 1986) and the majority of these will have suffered falls. The elderly are more likely to have suffered fractures and to have multiple injuries than young attenders (Burdett-Smith et al., 1989).

An important subgroup of injured fallers is those with head injuries. People of 65+ make up 10–15 per cent of admissions to hospital because of head injuries, and about three-quarters of these injuries are caused by falls and domestic accidents, compared to less than 35 per cent of the under 65s (Pentland et al., 1986). Likelihood of death in those with moderate or severe head injury (as judged by Glasgow Coma Scale score after resuscitation) is much higher in the elderly, and hospital stays for head-injured elderly are much longer than for younger patients, especially for mild or moderate injury. Functional outcome is frequently poor. 'A minor head injury is often the event that signals the end of independent living for the elderly man or woman living alone' (Pentland et al., 1986). Because more old people live alone, admission to hospital is more often necessary, even for those with minor injury, and the fact that the fall may have occurred because of illness complicates management. Over three quarters of the elderly admitted to hospital because of head injury have concurrent medical problems (Roy et al., 1986).

Psychological consequences

A fall is a potentially devastating thing to happen to an elderly person. The psychological impact of falling can be profound and has a number of facets. There is the effect of actual or potential injury and its implication for future physical functioning. A fall may increase the faller's feeling of vulnerability, particularly if he/she lives alone: 'What would happen if I fell again and wasn't able to get up on my own?'

The majority of people, as they age, internalise the negative view of the old that is prevalent in our society (French, 1990). The elderly are seen as physically and mentally decrepit, prone to instability, incontinence and senility. The occurrence of one of these attributes is seen as 'the beginning of the end', the onset of the feared mental and physical deterioration. The feeling that the body is no longer reliable shakes self-confidence to the core. Fear of further falls is a common sequel, and may be so debilitating as to stop the faller walking at all.

Fear of falling is a widespread problem for many elderly people, and is as common as falls themselves. Although fallers are more likely to be frightened of further falls, up to a third of non-fallers limit their activity because of fear of falling (Downton and Andrews, 1990). Several descriptions have been published of old people who suffered such severe anxiety and fear of further falling that they were unable to walk (Bhala et al., 1982; Murphy and Isaacs, 1982), and it has been suggested that symptoms of this severity might be a variant of agoraphobia. A 'post-fall' syndrome has been described, including features of alarm, hesitancy, irregularity of progress and a tendency to clutch and grab when asked to walk. Mortality amongst those who developed the 'post-fall syndrome' such that they were unable to walk independently was much higher than amongst those who did not (Murphy and Isaacs, 1982). The relationship between previous psychological function and the development of such inhibitory fear has not been studied.

Many elderly limit themselves to their houses, fearing to go out. Fear of falling is one of the reasons for this, and although the problem is not usually labelled agoraphobia, it shares some of the features of agoraphobia in younger people. There are often elements of anxiety and depression, and elderly fallers often mention that they are afraid of appearing physically incompetent in front of strangers. Like agoraphobics, they may severely restrict their activities, but even if true agoraphobia is not present, fear of falling and consequent anxiety and depression may lead to social withdrawal and reduction in activity. Paradoxically, this may in fact increase risk of falling because of the deterioration in general physical fitness that ensues.

The relationship between anxiety, depression and falling is a fascinating one, which is only beginning to be unravelled. A fairly high level of depressive symptoms has been shown in subjects shortly after hip fracture but it is not clear whether such symptoms were present prior to the fracture (Billig et al., 1986). Elderly people who have had falls are significantly more anxious and depressed than non-fallers, and although there is as yet little prospective information indicating the direction of causation, there is some evidence to suggest that it is falling itself which produces psychological distress. A prospective study of factors associated with falling in community elderly found a small increase in relative risk for those who were depressed (relative risk 1.7, 95 per cent CI 1.2–2.3), though cognitive impairment was a greater risk factor, as was sedative use (Tinetti et al., 1988). There seem to be two groups of fallers; physically frail, cognitively impaired and immobile elderly who tend to fall indoors; and fit, healthy, active elderly who fall whilst outdoors. However, both groups of fallers have high levels of anxiety and depression, suggesting that the falls may cause the psychological disturbance (Downton and Andrews, 1990).

Psychological factors may increase risk of falling. Elderly people with significant depression may be predisposed to falling because of associated psychomotor changes. Depressed patients have changes in gait compared to non-depressed control subjects, walking more slowly, with less propulsion and shorter stride length (Sloman et al., 1982). They may well be less aware of environmental hazards because of preoccupation with depressive thoughts, and may even consciously or subconsciously court danger as a form of 'indifferent suicide' (Lawton, 1967).

The response of family and friends to the elderly faller may compound rather than alleviate the problem. Quite naturally, a fall may provoke anxieties in the carer as well as the faller, but the commonest response is to limit the faller's activities and independence. Pressure may be put on the faller to go into residential care 'where there will be someone to help you if you fall again'. If admission to hospital has occurred, difficulties may be put in the way of health care staff attempting to arrange discharge home because of unreasonable demands that all risk of further falls be removed. It should not be forgotten that in a few individuals falls may be used as an attention-seeking device or a way of manipulating carers, either deliberately or subconsciously (Belfield et al., 1987).

It is an interesting point that although some elderly fallers are profoundly affected by having had one or more falls, others seem to accept the fact of falling with equanimity, not considering it necessary to interfere with their lifestyle or to report falling to any helping agency. Presumably, personality factors and psychological makeup have something to do with this, but further assessment of this group might reveal coping strategies that would help their more anxious peers.

Dependency

As already mentioned, falls and fear of falling seem to lead to old people restricting their activity (Vellas et al., 1987), or to their activity being restricted by carers. More specifically, increased dependency following one of the consequences of falling (fractured neck of femur) has been consistently found in a number of studies (Jensen and Bagger, 1982; Campbell, 1976). There is anecdotal evidence that falling itself leads to increased dependency (Gibson, 1987), and the possible mechanisms for this have already been discussed.

Falls and hospital admission

Falls are common reasons for elderly people to be admitted to hospital, both as an emergency and for investigation of recurrent falls. The presentation can be one of a number of situations – a single fall, with or without injury, recurrent falls, 'found on the floor', 'found collapsed', blackouts, dizzy spells, failure to cope at home, and so on. The large number of factors which may cause falls or predispose to falling means that the medical problems involved cover the whole spectrum of clinical practice. Falling is recognised to be one of the 'geriatric giants', a non-specific presentation of acute ill-health in the elderly, therefore potentially signifying any acute medical emergency. How frequently falls result in hospital admission, and the proportion of admissions of elderly people that are due to falls has, however, rarely been studied, unlike the frequency of falls once an elderly person is in hospital, and there is little reliable information. It is likely that at least a quarter of medical admissions in the elderly follow a fall or falls (Naylor and Rosin, 1970).

Information about elderly people attending Accident Departments in the UK following accidents at home (including falls), has been available since 1976 from the Home Accident Surveillance System (HASS). Information is

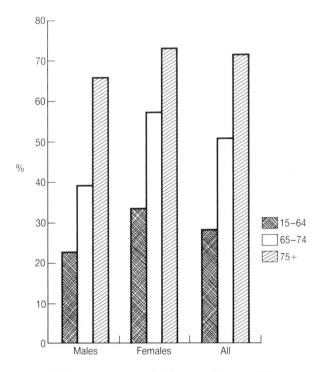

Fig. 2.3 Falls as a percentage of all home accidents at different ages
data from HASS, 1988

collected from people attending Accident Departments at a sample of hospitals in England and Wales, and more recently in Scotland and Northern Ireland as well (Consumer Safety Unit, 1988). In 1988, falls accounted for 28 per cent of home accidents in those aged 15–64, 51 per cent in those aged 65–74, and 72 per cent in those aged 75+ (Fig. 2.3). Estimates have been made from these data that approximately 200 000 people over 60 are treated at a hospital per year following a fall at home, with a rate of such falls of approximately 20 per 1000 of the population aged 60+. The elderly are more likely to be admitted to hospital from the Accident Department following a fall, and the proportion is greater in the 'old' elderly (75+) than the 'young elderly' (Fig. 2.4). Hip fractures alone accounted for 43 000 discharges and deaths in 1985 in England and Wales (HMSO, 1989). In the United States, there were 150 000 admissions for hip fracture in 1970, and these have been increasing at approximately 9 per cent per year (Devito et al., 1988).

People aged 65 and over attending Accident Departments following a home accident are almost ten times more likely to be admitted to hospital than younger adults, and once admitted, spend longer in hospital (Fig. 2.5). Almost all of those staying in hospital more than two weeks after an accident at home are over 65 (Fig. 2.6).

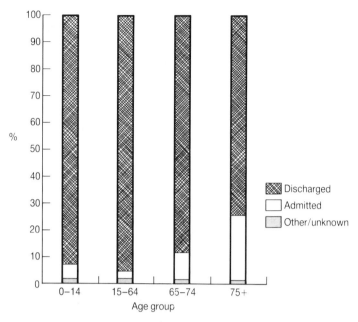

Fig. 2.4 Outcome after attendance at Accident and Emergency Department following a home accident
data from HASS, 1988

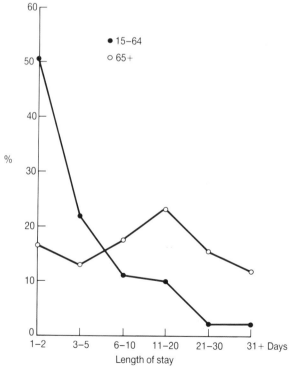

Fig. 2.5 Length of inpatient stay following a home accident
data from HASS, 1988

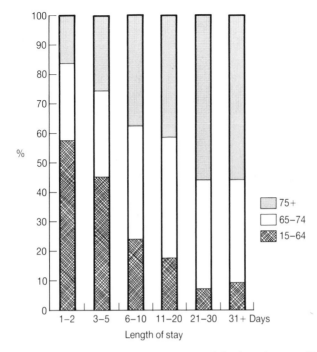

%

Fig. 2.6 Length of inpatient stay by age group following a home accident data from HASS, 1988

Falls and entry into institutional care

Although, as discussed above, it is likely that the occurrence of falls would be one of the factors that might lead to an elderly person entering residential care, little information is available about how frequently this happens. Risk of falling is a major cause of anxiety to carers, and a French study found that 39 per cent of 295 people aged 70+ who had fallen but suffered no serious injury were institutionalised at their families' request (Albarede and Vellas, 1985, quoted in Askham et al., 1990). In over 40 per cent of admissions to nursing homes in the United States frequent falls were mentioned as at least one of the reasons (Tinetti, 1985). If the faller suffers significant injury, the likelihood of returning to an independent existence is reduced, and entry into institutional care is more likely.

Economic consequences of falls

There are a number of components of the financial cost of falling, and because information systems are incomplete and often inaccurate it is very difficult to estimate the cost to health care services of falls amongst the elderly. Initial hospitalisation for acute care on medical, surgical or ortho-paedic wards often needs to be followed by a period of rehabilitation which can sometimes be prolonged, and a proportion of fallers will need continuing care of some kind. Outpatient and community care may be needed for those with lesser medical consequences of their fall, and the indirect costs because of informal carers who support elderly fallers rather than undertake paid employment are impossible to estimate. Some would argue that against these costs should be set the savings accrued by death of some fallers who no longer require payments from the public purse for health and social care.

Because of the demographic shifts in population in most countries, such economic consequences are likely to become more important. Population projections suggest that the largest proportional increase over the next 20–25 years will be in those aged 80 and over, the section of the elderly population most prone to falls and their complications. In addition, the relative decrease of younger adults and the greater entry into the workforce of women will mean that those providing informal care for the frail elderly will decrease, putting more pressure on hospital and community care providers. In order that this potential increase in demand should not swamp health and social care providers it is important to plan service provision appropriately, and to manage the health problems of the very elderly as expertly as possible to maximise their health and independence. Management of falls is an important component of this.

References

Askham, J., Glucksman, E., Owens, P., Swift, C., Tinker, A. and Yu, G. (1990). *A Review of Research on Falls Among Elderly People*. London, Age Concern Institute of Gerontology.

Belfield, P.W., Young, J.B., Bagnall, W.E. and Mulley, G.P. (1987). Deliberate falls in the elderly. *Age Ageing*. **16:** 123–124.

Berfenstam, R., Lagerberg, D. and Smedby, B. (1969). Victim characteristics in fatal home accidents. *Acta Socio-med Scand*. **1:** 145–164.

Bhala, R.P., O'Donnell, J. and Thoppil, E. (1982). Ptophobia. Phobic fear of falling and its clinical management. *Phys Ther*. **62:** 187–190.

Billig, N., Ahmed, S.W., Kenmore, P., Amaral, D. and Shakhashiri, M.Z. (1986). Assessment of depression and cognitive impairment after hip fracture. *J Am Geriatr Soc*. **34:** 499–503.

Burdett-Smith, P., Rowland, K., Woodhouse, K.W. and Maitra, A.K. (1989). A comparative study of the injury profile of the elderly patients in an accident and emergency department. *Arch Emerg Med*. **6:** 189–192.

Campbell, A.J. (1976). Femoral neck fractures in elderly women: a prospective study. *Age Ageing*. **5:** 102–109.

Campbell, A.J., Borrie, M.J., Spears, G.F., Jackson, S.L., Brown, J.S. and Fitzgerald, J.L. (1990). Circumstances and consequences of falls experienced by a community population 70 years and over during a prospective study. *Age Ageing*. **19:** 136–141.

Campbell, A.J., Diep, C., Reinken, J. and McCosh, L. (1985). Factors predicting mortality in a total population sample of the elderly. *J Epidemiol Comm Health*. **39:** 337–342.

Consumer Safety Unit (1988). *Home and Leisure Accident Research*.

Devito, C.A., Lambert, D.A., Sattin, R.W., Bacchelli, S., Ros, A. and Rodriguez,

J.G. (1988). Fall injuries among the elderly. Community based surveillance. *J Am Geriatr Soc*. **36:** 1029–1035.

Dove, A.F. and Dave, S.H. (1986). Elderly patients in the accident department and their problems. *Br Med J*. **292:** 807–809.

Downton, J.H. and Andrews, K. (1990). Postural disturbance and psychological symptoms amongst elderly people living at home. *Int J Geriatr Psychiatry*. **5:** 93–98.

Downton, J.H. and Andrews, K. (1991). Prevalence, characteristics and factors associated with falls among the elderly living at home. *Aging*. **3:** 219–228.

Eddy, T.P. (1973). Deaths from falls and fractures. Comparison of mortality in Scotland and United States with that in England and Wales. *Br J Prev Soc Med*. **27:** 247–254.

Fife, D. and Rappaport, E. (1987). What role do injuries play in the deaths of old people? *Accid Anal Prev*. **19:** 225–230.

French, S. (1990). Ageism. *Physiotherapy*. **76:** 178–182.

Gabell, A., Simons, M.A. and Nayak, U.S.L. (1985). Falls in the healthy elderly: predisposing causes. *Ergonomics*. **28:** 965–975.

Gibson, M.J. (1987). The prevention of falls in later life. A report of the Kellogg International Workgroup on the Prevention of Falls by the Elderly. *Dan Med Bull*. **Supplement No 4:** 5.

Grisso, J.A., Schwarz, D.F., Wishner, A.R., Weene, B., Holmes, J.H. and Sutton, R.L. (1990). Injuries in an elderly inner-city population. *J Am Geriatrics Soc*. **38:** 1326–1331.

Gryfe, C.I., Amies, A. and Ashley, M.J. (1977). A longitudinal study of falls in an elderly population. I: Incidence and morbidity. *Age Ageing*. **6:** 201–210.

HMSO (1989). *Hospital In-patient Enquiry: in-patient and day case trends 1979–1985*.

Hogue, C.C. (1982). Injury in late life. Part 1. Epidemiology. *J Am Geriatr Soc*. **30:** 183–190.

Jensen, J.S. and Bagger, J. (1982). Long term social prognosis after hip fractures. *Acta Orthop Scand*. **53:** 97–101.

Lawton, A.H. (1967). Accidental injuries to the aged and their psychologic impact. *Mayo Clin Proc*. **42:** 685–697.

Lucht, U. (1971). A prospective study of accidental falls and resulting injuries in the home among elderly people. *Acta Socio-Med Scand*. **3:** 105–120.

Melton, L.J. and Riggs, B.L. (1987). Epidermiology of age-related fractures. In: *The Osteoporotic Syndrome*, (ed.) Alvioli, L.V. Grune & Stratton, New York.

Morfitt, J.M. (1983). Falls in old people at home: intrinsic versus environmental factors in causation. *Public Health*. **97:** 115–120.

Murphy, J. and Isaacs, B. (1982). The post-fall syndrome. A study of 36 elderly patients. *Gerontology*. **28:** 265–270.

Naylor, R. and Rosin, A.J. (1970). Falling as a cause of admission to a geriatric unit. *Practitioner*. **205:** 327–330.

Oreskovich, M.R., Howard, J.D., Copass, M.K. and Carrico, C.J. (1984). Geriatric trauma: injury patterns and outcome. *J Trauma*. **24:** 565–572.

Pentland, B., Jones, P.A., Roy, C.W. and Miller, J.D. (1986). Head injury in the elderly. *Age Ageing*. **15:** 193–202.

Roy, C.W., Pentland, B. and Miller, J.D. (1986). The causes and consequences of minor head injury in the elderly. *Injury*. **17:** 220–223.

Sloman, L., Berridge, M., Homatidis, S., Hunter, D. and Duck, T. (1982). Gait patterns of depressed patients and normal subjects. *Am J Psychiatry*. **139:** 94–97.

Speechley, M. and Tinetti, M. (1991). Falls and injuries in frail and vigorous community elderly persons. *J Am Geriatr Soc*. **39:** 46–52.

Tinetti, M.E. (1985). Institutionalisation following falls. In Baker, S.P. and Harvey, A.H. (eds). Fall injuries in the elderly. *Clin Geriatr Med*. **1:** 501–508.

Tinetti, M.E., Speechley, M. and Ginter, S.F. (1988). Risk factors for falls among elderly persons living in the community. *N Engl J Med*. **319:** 1701–1707.

Vellas, B., Cayla, F., Bocquet, H., de Pemille, F. and Albarede, J.L. (1987). Prospective study of restriction of activity in old people after falls. *Age Ageing*. **16:** 189–193.

Wild, D., Nayak, U.S.L. and Isaacs, B. (1981). Prognosis of falls in old people at home. *J Epidemiol Comm Health*. **35:** 200–204.

Chapter 3 _____

Falls and fractures

Perhaps the most important consequence of a fall, both for the faller and for the community, is a fracture. Apart from the immediate pain and upset of the injury and the discomfort associated with treatment of the fracture, the longer term effects may be profound. Wrist and spinal fractures are probably the commonest fractures, but the economic and functional importance of hip fracture means that much more information is available about the management and consequences of this fracture. There is little doubt, however, that many fractures lead to prolonged and sometimes permanent reduction in function and independence.

Comparisons between studies of outcome after fractured neck of femur are hampered by different patient populations, different systems of care, and different definitions of mobility and independence. However, all demonstrate increased mortality compared to control populations (partly but not wholly explained by operative and in-hospital deaths), increase in functional dependence, and reduction in mobility after injury. Mortality after two and a half to three years is approximately 35 per cent (compared to an expected mortality of about 25 per cent) and actual and expected mortality curves do not become parallel until about five years post-fracture (Katz et al., 1967; Jensen and Bagger, 1982).

The exact degree to which mortality after hip fracture exceeds expected mortality varies depending on the pre-fracture level of health. In institutionalised, frail elderly one year mortality may be greater than 50 per cent, more than double that in similar non-fractured subjects, whereas in previously fit subjects living at home, one year mortality is between 12 and 20 per cent (Holmberg et al., 1986; Currie et al., 1986), which is at best only slightly greater than expected. It has been calculated that in the US, the annual mortality from hip fractures is 19 per 100 000 general population, constituting 2 per cent of total all-cause mortality, and a third of deaths attributable to accidents (Lewinnek et al., 1980). Mortality rates are higher in those with pre-existing medical problems and reduced independence. A more recent study of an unselected group of patients treated at a fairly typical English district general hospital showed a six-month mortality of 29 per cent, with only 50 per cent having returned to their normal place of residence at six months (Greatorex, 1988).

A quarter to a half of fractured neck of femur victims are more dependent a year after their injury than they were before (Katz et al., 1967; Thomas and Steven, 1974). Those who are admitted from their own homes tend to do better but the most important factors in successful rehabilitation appear to be general medical condition and age.

Relationship between falls and fractures

The proportion of falls that are reported to result in fractures varies depending on whether subjects are living at home or in institutional care, and also on the way in which information is collected. In elderly people living at home, fractures occur in less than 5 per cent of falls (Nevitt et al., 1989; Campbell et al., 1990) but are commoner in women than men and increase in frequency with increasing age. Amongst those in institutional care, there is a much wider spread of reported incidence, partly reflecting the different systems of monitoring falls and accidents. Some studies report a very high incidence of fracture in fallers, but this is likely to mean that falls without injury are under-reported. It seems probable, however, that broken bones following a fall are slightly commoner in institutionalised elderly than amongst those at home, reflecting the increased frailty of such populations.

Old people with fractures commonly give a history of recurrent falls prior to that resulting in their fracture (Johnell and Nilsson, 1985) and seem more likely to have fallen in the previous year than controls (Evans et al., 1979; Cook et al., 1982). Conversely, people having multiple falls may be less likely to suffer fractures and have a lower fracture rate per fall (Baker and Harvey, 1985).

Most fractures in the elderly result from falls. However, a fall is a necessary but not a sufficient cause of a fracture. Once a fall has occurred, the risk of fracture is related directly to trauma intensity and inversely to bone strength. Reduced bone strength (mostly due to osteoporosis) does not affect all elderly in an equal fashion, with women and the very elderly being disproportionately affected. This is mirrored by the incidence of fractures.

Unfortunately the relationship between osteoporosis and fractures is not entirely clear. Although those with osteoporosis are at greater risk of fractures than those without (Fig. 3.1), on a population level the difference between fracture patients and controls in degree of osteoporosis is small (Cummings, 1985). Most elderly women have lost sufficient bone for the hip to fracture with the impact of an unprotected fall, and although almost one woman in four living to the age of 90 in England can expect to suffer a hip fracture, three quarters will not. Differences in bone density between individual women are not great enough to discriminate between those who will and those who will not later suffer a fracture: this will be determined by

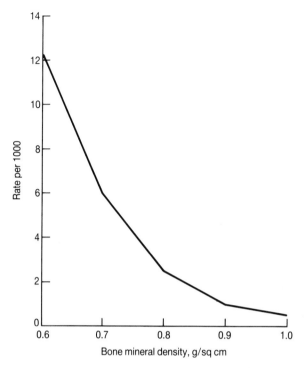

Fig. 3.1   Risk of intertrochanteric fractures for different bone mineral densities
after Melton & Riggs, 1987

chance, and by conditions that increase the risk of falling or cause loss of normal protective reflexes. Osteoporosis may, however, be more important in the aetiology of fractures in the 'young elderly' (Cooper et al., 1987; Eriksson and Lindgren, 1989).

Falls in the elderly are most often from a standing height or less, and these sorts of falls are the major causes of fractures in this age group, unlike fractures in young people which usually involve a greater trauma intensity (Fig. 3.2). The ability to absorb energy is important, and this depends on the integrated function of muscles, joints, ligaments and bone. There is a strong correlation between muscle strength and bone density (Eriksson and Lindgren, 1989), and effective muscle function helps to absorb the energy of a fall. In addition, the amount of adipose tissue is relevant. Oestrogen levels, which affect bone density, are higher in those with greater amounts of adipose tissue, because of peripheral conversion of adrenal hormones to oestrogen in fat, and it has also been suggested that 'well endowed subjects 'bounce' on adipose hips' thus preventing fracture (Boyce, 1987).

Neuromuscular reflexes are also important, both in preventing falls and in saving oneself from injury once a fall becomes inevitable. The fact that the incidence of fractures of the distal forearm peaks at about 60 years in women

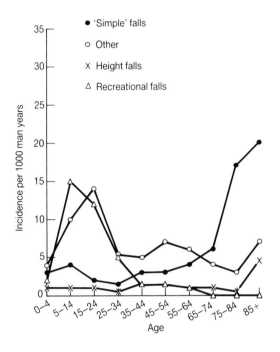

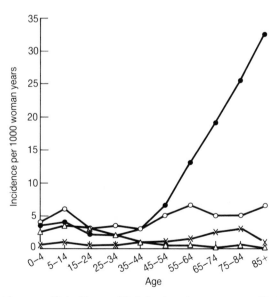

Fig. 3.2   Age- and sex-specific incidence of limb fractures by cause among Rochester, Minnesota residents, 1968–1971 (Melton & Riggs, 1985)

and then declines, unlike the incidence of proximal femoral fractures and falls themselves, is taken as evidence that with increasing age there is failure of protective reflexes to break a fall (Miller and Evans, 1985).

There has been much discussion about the relationship between physical activity, osteoporosis and fractures, and about the role of dietary calcium intake in causation and prevention of osteoporosis. As mentioned above, there is a relationship between osteoporosis and fractures but it is not very strong. Some work suggests that reduced calcium intake (which may accelerate osteoporosis) is not a risk factor for hip fracture (Wickham et al., 1989), though increased calcium intake may protect against fractures (Holbrook et al., 1988). The picture is complicated by the extremely variable absorption of calcium which can be as low as 15 per cent or as high as 60 per cent of an ingested load (Need et al., 1990). There is, however, a clear relationship between physical activity and both falls and femoral fractures. This is true both for activity during early and middle life (Astrom et al., 1987; Boyce and Vessey, 1988) and in older age (Wickham et al., 1989). It is thought that increased physical activity results in better general health as well as greater muscle strength, and that both these factors improve neuromuscular reflexes, protecting against falls as well as fractures.

Epidemiology of fractures

So-called age-related fractures (wrist, neck of femur and vertebral crush fractures) are common in Western countries, and a white European or North American woman has a lifetime risk of having such a fracture of 30 per cent, compared to a lifetime risk of 9 per cent for breast cancer. Those surviving into 'old' old age (80+) are at increasing risk of such fractures (Fig. 3.3). The

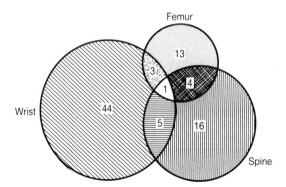

Fig. 3.3 Venn diagram illustrating the estimated frequency of wrist, femur and spine fracture in women aged 80. The areas of overlap give an estimate of the frequency with which two or three of these osteoporotic fractures occur in the same patient
from Peacock, 1985

incidence of many fractures increases exponentially with age and the vast majority of fractures in this age group are caused by falls (Melton and Riggs, 1987).

Figures from the Hospital In-patient Enquiry give some idea of the scale of the problem of health care provision for fracture patients in England (HMSO, 1989). In 1985 almost half of the average daily bed use in Trauma and Orthopaedics was by those aged 65 and over, and the majority of those beds would be used for injuries sustained in falls. Over 40 per cent of bed-days for fractures were for those with fractured neck of femur. In that year, 43 230 people were treated in hospital in England for fractured neck of femur, and virtually all of these would be elderly suffering their fracture as a result of a fall. Hip fracture patients accounted for almost a quarter of patients treated in hospital for a fracture.

There are some interesting features of the epidemiology of fractures which give tantalising glimpses of some of the possible causes. There is a marked difference in fracture incidence in different parts of the world, and between different races. For instance, whites have a higher hip fracture rate than blacks in the US, and white Europeans have higher rates than Asians.

Standardised comparisons of hip fracture incidence per total population in different countries give figures ranging from 5.6 per 100 000 in black South Africans, 42.8 per 100 000 in the UK, 69.6 per 100 000 in Sweden, to 98 per 100 000 in the US (Lewinnek et al., 1980). All these figures come from studies carried out in the 1960s and early 1970s. It is interesting that, apart from the South African figures, the incidence for men does not alter to a great extent from one part of the world to another, whilst that for women mainly accounts for the national differences. Theories to try to explain these differences have included effects of diet, latitude, physical activity, genetic differences and differing prevalence of osteoporosis. The incidence of proximal femoral fractures (and other fractures) rises with increasing age, and there is a tenfold difference in incidence between ages 65–69 and 90+ (Evans et al., 1979).

As well as absolute differences in incidence, there are different patterns of incidence. In Europe and the US, the typical picture is of an exponential increase in fractures of proximal femur, humerus and pelvis with age, which is much more marked in women than men (Fig. 3.4). Fractures of the proximal femur are most frequent, followed by proximal humerus, then pelvic fractures (Melton and Riggs, 1987). This exponential rise in proximal femoral fractures has been reported to begin in middle life in both men and women, with no change in rate of increase after the menopause (Hedlund et al., 1987), though other studies suggest that the rate in women increases post-menopausally. In Malaysia men seem to be more susceptible to proximal femoral fractures than women, though absolute incidence is less than in the West. Humeral fractures are, however, more common in Malaysian women than men (Wong, 1966).

As shown in Fig. 3.4, the pattern of distal forearm fracture (Colle's fracture) incidence differs from other fractures, in that incidence in women begins to rise at an earlier age and levels off in the 60s to 70s rather than

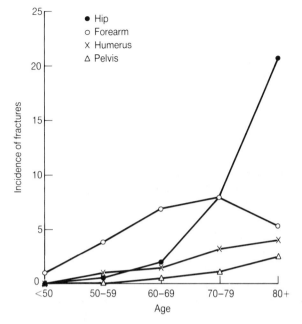

Fig. 3.4   Age-specific incidence rates (per 1000 women per year) of various fractures

continuing to increase as does incidence of the other 'age-related' fractures. Distal forearm fractures, although relatively 'trivial' compared with femoral fractures, do have significant impact on orthopaedic workload, making up 10–15 per cent of the caseload of fracture clinics (Miller and Evans, 1985).

There appears to have been a significant increase in incidence of proximal femoral fracture over the last few decades (Lewis, 1981; Hedlund et al., 1985), increasing at between 5 and 10 per cent per year, while the population at risk has increased by only 2 per cent per year. This increase, which also affects other fractures, may have begun to level off during the 1980s (Spector et al., 1990). Again, a number of hypotheses have been advanced to explain the increase in incidence, the most popular being the steady decline in physical activity, both at work and at home. However, it has also been argued that the improvement in general health of the elderly has increased risk of fracture because the elderly are *more* active (Finsen, 1988), and one study has shown a greater risk of fractures despite a lower risk of falls in vigorous as compared to frail elderly (Speechley and Tinetti, 1991).

Other patterns gleaned from fracture incidence are that in women, femoral fractures largely result from falls at home, whereas fractures of clavicle, radius, tibia and fibula are mainly caused by falls away from home. This pattern is not apparent in men (Knowelden et al., 1964). Women comprise 70–80 per cent of patients with hip fractures, and the average age is generally in the eighth decade. The majority of femoral fracture patients have concurrent medical illnesses (Campbell, 1976).

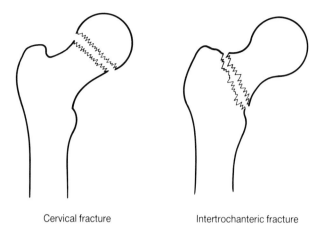

Cervical fracture   Intertrochanteric fracture

Fig. 3.5 Illustrations of cervical and trochanteric femoral fractures

Femoral fractures are either cervical or trochanteric (Fig. 3.5). The ratio of trochanteric to cervical fractures increases with age, and there is some evidence that trochanteric fractures occur in those with more advanced biological ageing. These patients have more concurrent disease and post-fracture management is more difficult, with delayed recovery and a greater likelihood of increased dependency (Lawton et al., 1983).

Estimates have been made of the financial implication of age-related fractures, and although giving a specific figure is probably meaningless, it clearly runs to billions of dollars annually (Baker and Harvey, 1985). With the apparent increase in incidence as well as the demographic increase in the very elderly, who are particularly at risk of fractures and who are more likely to need more prolonged rehabilitation, those costs are likely to increase. It has been estimated that if the current rates of hip fracture do not alter there will be an increase of 33 per cent in number of cases by 2016, and if the present rate of increase continues there will be an increase of 254 per cent by that date (Royal College of Physicians, 1989).

Risk factors for fractures

Risk factors for fractures fall into two main groups: those factors which reduce the strength of bone, and therefore its ability to resist breaking; and those factors which increase risk of falling. Risk of falling is discussed in more detail in Chapter 5. As has been mentioned above, in practice there is not a clear cut-off between those two areas, and factors which affect bone strength may also, through different mechanisms, alter risk of falling. The mechanisms by which particular factors increase risk of fracture is not always clear, and the associations may not necessarily denote causation, but may be linked via another factor or factors.

Age

The increased incidence of fractures in older people is partly due to increased risk of falling, and partly to decrease in bone strength, but neither fully explain the exponential increase in fractures with age (Melton and Riggs, 1985).

Sex

Women are much more prone to 'age-related' fractures than men. This is partly due to differences in bone mass and bone strength between the sexes, and women are somewhat more likely to fall than men. Once again, however, this does not seem to be the whole story, and does not explain why hip fracture incidence in women is two to three times that in men whereas Colles fractures and fractures of the proximal humerus and pelvis are 6–8 times commoner in women than men (Cummings et al., 1985).

Osteoporosis

Bone consists of two types, cortical and cancellous. Cortical bone is a compact layer which predominates in the shafts of long bones, and cancellous bone forms the interior meshwork of bones, particularly the vertebrae, pelvis and ends of long bones. The adult skeleton is about 80 per cent cortical and 20 per cent cancellous bone. In cancellous bone the trabeculae form an interconnecting lattice designed to resist mechanical loads. Osteoporosis affects both types of bone, but the effect of a decrease in bone mineral density on bone strength is more marked in cancellous bone because trabeculae may become discontinuous or even disappear, destroying the bone architecture and markedly impairing ability to withstand stress, so that risk of fracture increases disproportionately to the amount of bone lost. In addition, low rates of bone turnover impair the ability to repair fatigue damage and may thus increase the risk of fracture, independently of bone mineral density. These two facts may help to explain why studies have not always shown a clear relationship between bone density and fracture risk. There is probably also a threshold effect (Fig. 3.6), whereby bone strength is sufficient even if reduced, until a critical level is reached (Newton-John and Morgan, 1968).

There are a number of factors which have their effect on fracture incidence via an effect on bone strength and osteoporosis. Cigarette smoking is associated with a decrease in bone density, which may partly reflect the lower body weight of smokers, and smoking affects oestrogen levels in women. Dietary factors, particularly calcium intake, have an effect on osteoporosis. There is no clear evidence that increased calcium intake can reverse bone loss at the time of the menopause, but there is reasonable evidence that calcium supplementation can reduce the rate of bone loss and may prevent fractures

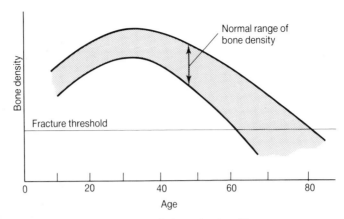

Fig. 3.6   Changes in bone density with age

(Need et al., 1990), and it has been argued that bone loss may actually be prevented by an adequate calcium intake (Heaney, 1990).

Drugs

Alcohol consumption affects fracture incidence partly because it predisposes to falls, though this is only a minor cause of falls in the elderly. Heavy drinkers have lower bone mineral density and more rapid bone loss than non-drinkers, perhaps because of the direct toxic effect of alcohol, perhaps because of associated poor nutrition. Any drug with a sedative effect increases risk of fracture because the impairment of alertness leads to a higher risk of falling.

Corticosteroids increase bone loss, and long term use is associated with osteoporosis and increased risk of fractures, though vertebral fractures are commoner than fractures at other sites. Excess thyroid hormone leads to osteoporosis, but replacement doses in those with hypothyroidism do not.

There has been much discussion about the effects of thiazide diuretics on hip fracture incidence. Thiazides may protect against fractures, probably because they reduce calcium loss in urine, though they also reduce intestinal absorption of calcium. Thiazides have been shown to increase bone mineral density (Wasnich et al., 1983) and there have been a number of studies demonstrating a protective effect of thiazides on hip fractures (Rashiq and Logan, 1986; Ray et al., 1989), but a recent case-control study did not find a protective effect of thiazides. There was a slight increase in risk of fracture with current use of a thiazide diuretic, though use of a loop diuretic increased risk of fracture to a greater extent (Heidrich et al., 1991).

Physical activity

It has been suggested that the increase in incidence of fractures over the last few decades is related to the decrease in physical activity of the population generally. Fewer people have physically demanding occupations, more people use cars rather than walking, and social activities tend to be more passive than in earlier years (for example, watching 'Come Dancing' on the television rather than going out dancing oneself).

Physical activity has effects on risk of fracture both because of effects of activity on bone mass and because low levels of activity may be associated with impaired protective mechanisms against falls (Hansson et al., 1982), possibly because of impaired muscle function (Aniansson et al., 1984). There is evidence that exercise programmes increase bone density in young and elderly subjects, and that elderly people who exercise regularly have higher bone density than their sedentary peers (Schapira, 1988). It has been estimated that regular exercise would reduce the risk of hip fracture by at least half (Law et al., 1991). Physical activity in middle life may be as important as level of activity in old age in maintaining bone mass and limiting osteoporosis.

Nutrition

The relationship between nutrition and fractures is a complex one. As discussed above, there is some evidence that dietary factors, particularly calcium intake and alcohol consumption, affect bone mineral density, and thus may affect fracture incidence. Poor overall nutritional state may increase fracture incidence by increasing liability to fall, especially during cold weather, and certainly seems to affect outcome following hip fracture (Bastow et al., 1983).

Management of the elderly fracture patient

Acute management

The immediate management of an elderly patient with a fracture has a number of important aspects, which can be considered under the following headings.

Resuscitation
With anything other than a minor distal fracture an elderly patient with a broken bone has a potentially major injury. This may be associated with significant blood loss and shock, with important physiological responses to trauma and with potential effects on fluid balance, thermoregulation and homoeostasis generally. Because one of the important aspects of ageing is loss

of reserve and impaired ability to cope with physiological stress, resuscitation is potentially more important and needs to be carried out even more swiftly than in younger patients with similar degrees of injury. In addition, homoeostatic responses may be impaired by the fallers regular medication, such as betablockers for ischaemic heart disease or hypertension, diuretics, corticosteroids, and so on. Resuscitation may particularly be required if there has been a 'long lie' (that is if the injured person has been unable to get up unassisted for a period of an hour or more), if there is more than one fracture, or if there has been much blood loss from the fracture site. The effects of concurrent medical problems may need to be taken into account. As part of resuscitation, prompt admission and management of injuries is important. There is no excuse for compounding the problems of the injury by leaving the patient on a hard trolley in a cold Accident and Emergency Department waiting for a bed on an orthopaedic ward.

Diagnosis of the injury

This is usually fairly straightforward unless facilities for radiographs are not available, but a number of important questions should be considered as well as which bone is broken. Is there more than one fracture? Are there other non-fracture injuries? Are there associated soft tissue injuries? Are there any neurological injuries (diagnostic difficulties may be encountered because of age-related neurological changes or pre-existing neurological disease)? Does the type of fracture imply particular types of management?

Cause of the fall

This should always be considered at an early stage, because of the possibility that the fall occurred because of acute illness (e.g. infection, myocardial infarction, stroke) which may affect decisions about management of the fracture(s). It is probably true to say that most elderly with femoral fractures, particularly the very elderly (80+), have fallen because they are ill.

Deciding on appropriate treatment and preparing the patient for treatment

The current consensus of opinion is that operative treatment is the most appropriate management of fractured neck of femur, and that early operation gives the best chance of good recovery. If the alternative is a long period of immobilisation, operation for fractures at other sites may also reduce long-term morbidity. Decisions about treatment may need to be made by orthopaedic surgeons in conjunction with anaesthetists and geriatricians. In general the standard management for fractures such as hip fractures should be immediate operation with early postoperative mobilisation if at all possible, and surgical treatment should be postponed only for very clear and over-riding reasons. For fractures which do not require immediate surgical treatment, such as humerus or pelvis, the aim should be to provide sufficient analgesia to allow early mobilisation. Prolonged periods of immobilisation are almost always devastating for frail elderly people, who risk succumbing to the complications of bed rest (Harper and Lyles, 1988). The best options to aim for are immediate operation and early mobilisation, local immobilisation followed by early mobilisation, or analgesia and early mobilisation, as appropriate for the type of fracture.

It is perhaps fair to say that orthopaedic surgeons and anaesthetists do not always see the late effects of non-operative treatment, as such patients tend to be transferred to the care of geriatricians for long term management, which may explain why geriatricians are sometimes more keen to subject the patient to operation than are anaesthetists or orthopaedic surgeons. Deciding not to operate may save a patient from dying on the operating table, but in exchange may result in a prolonged state of pain, ill-health and dependency. In these situations surgery may be justified despite a high operative risk, but careful discussion may be needed with the patient and relatives for proper informed consent to be obtained.

Avoiding complications of the fracture and its management
The complications of the fracture (blood loss, infection, fat embolism, non-union, etc.) are covered in standard orthopaedic texts, and their management will not be considered here. The complications of the management of the fracture are equally important, and many result from immobilisation. The complications of bed rest are legion, but the most important to be considered initially are the development of pressure sores, deep venous thrombosis and impaired bladder and bowel function.

Pressure sores occur with depressing and predictable regularity in elderly fracture patients, and 50 per cent or more of those with hip fractures develop sores over the sacrum or heels (Royal College of Physicians, 1989). The effects of the injury and the physiological responses to stress make the development of pressure sores more likely. The vast majority of these pressure sores could be prevented by assessment (using one of the several risk scores available, such as the Norton or Waterlow scores, Table 3.1) to pick out those at highest risk, and more importantly, by provision of pressure relieving devices to those at risk at the time of admission, *before* a pressure sore has developed. Pressure relieving mattresses should be widely available in Accident Departments. It is unfortunate that the tissue damage causing deep pressure sores often occurs some time before the sore becomes apparent, which means that the connection between cause and effect is not always clear. There is some logic in providing some form of pressure relief to sacrum and heels to all patients with hip fracture from the moment of admission, and this is likely to be cost effective given the estimated extra cost of healing pressure sores, which runs into tens of thousands of pounds (Hibbs, 1988).

Deep vein thrombosis following fractures, particularly hip fractures, is common and almost certainly under-diagnosed. It is now clear that prophylaxis, using low dose subcutaneous heparin, is effective and does not significantly increase operative bleeding or wound healing.

Table 3.1 Risk scores for development of pressure sores
(a) The Waterlow pressure sore prevention/treatment policy.

(Ring scores in table, add total. Several scores per category can be used.)		
Build/weight for height	Average	0
	Above average	1
	Obese	2
	Below average	3
Continence	Complete/catheterised	0
	Occasionally incontinent	1
	Catheterised + incontinent faeces	2
	Doubly incontinent	3
Skin type		
Visual risk areas	Healthy	0
	Tissue paper	1
	Dry	1
	Oedematous	1
	Clammy (temp.)	1
	Discoloured	2
	Broken/spot	3
Mobility	Fully	0
	Restless/fidgety	1
	Apathetic	2
	Restricted	3
	Inert/traction	4
	Chair-bound	5
Sex and age	Male	1
	Female	2
	14–49	1
	50–64	2
	65–74	3
	75–80	4
	81+	5
Appetite	Average	0
	Poor	1
	NG tube/fluids only	2
	Nil by mouth/anorexic	3
Special risks		
Tissue malnutrition	e.g. Terminal cachexia	8
	Cardiac failure	5
	Peripheral vascular disease	5
	Anaemia	2
	Smoking	1
Neurological deficit	e.g. Diabetes, MS, CVA	
	Motor/sensory loss, paraplegia	4–6
Major surgery/trauma	Orthopaedic-below waist, spinal	5
	On table >2 hours	5
Medication	Steroids, cytotoxics, high-dose anti-inflammatory drugs	4
Score	10+ At Risk	
	15+ High Risk	
	20+ Very High Risk	

(b) The Norton pressure sore risks assessment scoring system.

General condition	Mental state	Activity	Mobility	Incontinence
4. Good	4. Alert	4. Ambulant	4. Full	4. Not
3. Fair	3. Apathetic	3. Walks with help	3. Slightly limited	3. Occasional
2. Poor	2. Confused	2. Chair-bound	2. Very limited	2. Usually/urine
1. Very bad	1. Stuperose	1. Bedfast	1. Immobile	1. Doubly

Note: A total score of 14 or below means that the patient is at high risk.

Bladder and bowel function are not seen as exciting therapeutic challenges, but are crucially important for the patient's self-esteem, and often affect discharge plans to an inordinate degree. Many fracture patients who are treated surgically are catheterised in the operative or immediate postoperative stages and are thus liable to the interference with continence that this often produces. In addition, if they are immobilised they have to rely on assistance from nursing staff for toileting. Many elderly people have a degree of urinary urgency, and in the absence of prompt assistance may be incontinent. This can be devastating to morale. The problem may be compounded by the almost invariable development of constipation, largely related to immobility, fluid depletion and poor nutritional intake.

An important complication of the initial post-injury phase is disturbance of fluid balance. Although a proportion of old people have normal renal function, it is safest to assume that elderly patients have some degree of renal impairment, and the majority have difficulty coping with fluid depletion. Conversely, because of the hormonal response to injury, fracture patients generally are also less able to cope with fluid overload. It is, however, much more common in practice for the fracture patient to be under-hydrated than over-hydrated. This leads to hypovolaemia, which worsens renal function, predisposes to venous thrombosis, and increases risk of pressure sores.

Impaired thermoregulation may have played a part in the fall, as elderly people with abnormal metabolic responses to a cold environment who become hypothermic develop incoordination, predisposing to falls, but once an injury has taken place, thermoregulation is very likely to be disordered, with a drop in skin and core temperature and interference with normal thermoregulatory responses (Little and Stoner, 1981). Maintaining normal body temperature, and preventing a drop in temperature in the early stages following injury and surgery can reduce protein breakdown (Carli and Itiaba, 1986), and, at least theoretically, speed recovery.

A proportion of elderly patients with fractures will be poorly nourished, and their outcome is likely to be significantly worse (Bastow et al., 1983). In addition, many ill old people in hospital do not eat enough to provide adequate nutrition, and as post injury intake is mainly governed by previous eating habits rather than present requirements, those who are already malnourished will tend to become more so. There is now some evidence that nutritional supplementation can improve recovery in the short and longer term (Delmi et al., 1990), and consideration should be given to supplementary feeding, particularly in those with overtly poor nutritional state.

Dealing with concurrent illnesses

Not all elderly people taking diuretics have heart failure, and not all those taking antihypertensives have true hypertension. However, some do, so medications and the indications for taking them should be critically reviewed. Previously undiagnosed conditions may also require treatment, but first need diagnosis! Although most elderly people are physically well, mentally clear and independent, those with falls are more likely to be physically and mentally frail than non-fallers, and the presence of underlying illness(es) should be carefully considered as their presence may affect management of the fracture and rehabilitation once the fracture has been treated.

Medical management of an elderly person

The characteristic feature of the elderly is that they have reduced reserve. As mentioned above they are less able to cope with homoeostatic stresses than younger people. Symptoms and signs of disease may also be masked. These factors must be considered at all stages of management, and are particularly important with respect to fluid balance, renal function and cardiovascular function.

There are a number of pointers to patients at risk (Table 3.2), and the presence of one or more of them should alert medical and nursing staff to potential problems, both in the early stages of management of the injury and later, during rehabilitation. Because of the difficulty of assessing some elderly patients, it is sensible to check full blood count, urea, creatinine and electrolytes, and possibly chest X-ray in most, if not all, elderly fracture patients, even if the injury is apparently trivial. It is probably also sensible to recheck blood count and urea and electrolytes a couple of days postoperatively to pick up those who are running into problems with renal function (usually because of inadequate fluid input and/or hypotension postoperatively) and those whose blood loss has not been adequately replenished.

Table 3.2 Indicators of patients at risk of medical complications following a fracture.

Multiple medications
'Biologically old'
Multiple chronic health problems
Pre-fall immobility and/or dependence
Cognitive impairment
Fall because of acute illness
Evidence of organ impairment on simple investigation

Rehabilitation following fracture

Rehabilitation should begin as soon as the injury occurs, and appropriate management of the fracture is clearly an important part of this. So, too, is diagnosis and treatment of concurrent medical problems and prevention of avoidable complications of injury such as pressure sores and faecal impaction. There often seems to be a 'window of opportunity' for rehabilitation, which may be missed if patients have to wait for long periods for transfer to specific 'rehabilitation units'.

Successful rehabilitation of patients following fractures is little different from rehabilitation following any other illness or injury in elderly people. It depends on a positive attitude of mind amongst staff, and a coordinated approach with each member of the multidisciplinary team respecting and making use of the skills of the others for the benefit of the patient. Because nurses spend 24 hours a day with the patient they are the key members of the team, and the success of rehabilitation largely depends on them. If nursing staff on an orthopaedic ward have an enlightened and positive view of managing elderly patients, then the atmosphere of the ward is likely to promote independence and speed rehabilitation. Support and interest from medical staff will help to maintain this atmosphere. Adequate numbers of nursing staff are vital for providing a good standard of care and maintaining staff morale, and there is evidence that where nursing and other staff levels are low, outcome is worse (Evans et al., 1980). When staffing levels are inadequate, there is a tendency to do things for patients rather than encouraging them to do things for themselves – promoting independence is time-consuming.

The role of physiotherapists is clearly important, as regaining mobility is usually an early stage in regaining independence. It may be necessary to work on balance first, particularly if the initial treatment of the injury has been complicated and required a period of bed rest. Advice may be required on appropriate walking aids, and correct techniques of standing and transferring. Close liaison with nursing staff is important so that every requirement to stand, transfer and walk during the course of the day and night is used as an opportunity to practice and consolidate new skills. If time and staff numbers permit, teaching the patient to get up from the floor safely in the event of further falls can help the patient to regain confidence (see Chapter 7).

The occupational therapist has an important role in assessing the patients abilities in 'activities of daily living', practising the required skills with the patient and assessing the home circumstances prior to discharge from hospital. In combination with the social worker, an assessment can be made of requirements for community support after discharge. The social worker also has a role in counselling the patient and relatives, particularly where either has unrealistic expectations about the risk of further falls.

Orthogeriatric liaison

Because the majority of patients with fractured neck of femur (and a substantial proportion of patients with other fractures) are elderly and often ill, an orthopaedic surgeon needs either to become a geriatrician him/herself or enlist the help of geriatricians to manage such patients optimally. In particular, some sort of rehabilitation is needed for a proportion of elderly patients with fractures. For this reason a number of different schemes providing liaison between orthopaedic and geriatric departments have been set up in the UK. In some areas there is no specific liaison and patients are referred to geriatricians on an *ad hoc* basis once it becomes clear that their progress is slow. Some hospitals have a specific geriatric/orthopaedic unit with transfer of most patients at an early stage. Others have a separate rehabilitation unit for 'difficult' cases, and many more patients with more straightforward problems receive their rehabilitation on the acute orthopaedic unit and are discharged directly from there. In a few places there are schemes for very early discharge and rehabilitation at home for a proportion of fractured neck of femur patients (Pryor et al., 1988).

In the USA the situation is affected by the question of funds for care. For those dependent on Medicare, a quarter to a half of hip fracture rehabilitation is carried out in skilled nursing facilities (Bonar et al., 1990). There is some evidence, however, that the lack of coordinated geriatric/orthopaedic rehabilitation services in the US results in slower recovery of patients with fractured neck of femur.

The Royal College of Physicians, in their report on the management of fractured neck of femur (1989), has proposed a model operating policy for combined management of hip fracture between orthopaedic and geriatric departments (Fig. 3.7). What is achievable depends on the local availability and distribution of resources and the interests of individual geriatricians and orthopaedic surgeons, but with cooperation and goodwill between the two departments much can be accomplished for the benefit of the patients. That cooperation should be a two-way process, however. Orthopaedic surgeons who expect their geriatrician colleagues merely to provide a dumping ground for difficult patients, without providing orthopaedic input where necessary to the rehabilitation process will not get the best from them. Geriatricians who have to fight what sometimes feels like a fight to the death (of the patient, usually) to persuade orthopaedic surgeons to reoperate, for example where pain from displacement of fracture fixation is resulting in failure to mobilise, will eventually lose their desire to cooperate.

A personal list of areas where a geriatrician can be of assistance in the management of elderly fracture patients would include the following: medical assessment of those who have fallen because of acute or chronic illness, and medical management of complications of injury or treatment; advice about when, and sometimes whether to operate, and advice about when to stop treating (usually in those who are clearly not going to survive); post-injury

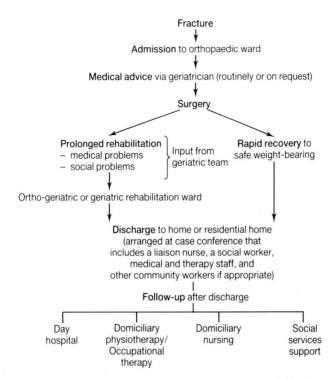

Fig. 3.7 A model operating policy for combined management of hip fracture between orthopaedic and geriatric departments (Royal College of Physicians, 1989)

rehabilitation; and aiding development of rehabilitation environment on the orthopaedic ward.

References

Aniansson, A., Zetterberg, C., Hedberg, M. and Henriksson, K.G. (1984). Impaired muscle function with aging. A background factor in the incidence of fractures of the proximal end of the femur. *Clin Orth Rel Res.* **191:** 193–201.

Astrom, J., Ahnqvist, S., Beertema, J. and Jonsson, B. (1987). Physical activity in women sustaining fractures of the neck of the femur. *J Bone Joint Surg.* **69B:** 381–383.

Baker, S.P. and Harvey, A.H. (1985). Fall injuries in the elderly. *Clin Geriatr Med.* **1:** 501–508.

Bastow, M.D., Rawlings, J. and Allison, S.P. (1983). Undernutrition, hypothermia, and injury in elderly women with fractured femur: an injury response to altered metabolism? *Lancet.* **1:** 143–146.

Bonar, S.K., Tinetti, M.E., Speechley, M. and Cooney, L.M. (1990). Factors associated with short- versus long-term skilled nursing facility placement among community-living hip fracture patients. *J Am Geriatr Soc.* **38:** 1139–1144.

Boyce, W.J. (1987). Osteoporosis, falls and age in fracture of the proximal femur (letter). *Br Med J.* **295:** 444–445.

Boyce, W.J. and Vessey, M.P. (1988). Habitual physical inertia and other factors in relation to risk of fracture of the proximal femur. *Age Ageing.* **17:** 319–327.

Campbell, A.J. (1976). Femoral neck fractures in elderly women: a prospective study. *Age Ageing.* **5:** 102–109.

Campbell, A.J., Borrie, M.J., Spears, G.F., Jackson, S.L., Brown, J.S. and Fitzgerald, J.L. (1990). Circumstances and consequences of falls experienced by a community population 70 years and over during a prospective study. *Age Ageing.* **19:** 136–141.

Carli, F. and Itiaba, K. (1986). Effect of heat conservation during and after major abdominal surgery on muscle protein breakdown in elderly patients. *Br J Anaesth.* **58:** 502–507.

Cook, P.J., Exton-Smith, A.N., Brocklehurst, J.C. and Lempert-Barber, S.M. (1982). Fractured femurs, falls and bone disorders. *J Roy Coll Phys Lond.* **16:** 45–49.

Cooper, C., Barker, D.J., Morris, J. and Briggs, R.S. (1987). Osteoporosis, falls and age in fracture of the proximal femur. *Br Med J.* **295:** 13–15.

Cummings, S.R. (1985). Are patients with hip fractures more osteoporotic? A review of the evidence. *Am J Med.* **78:** 487–494.

Cummings, S.R., Kelsey, J.L., Nevitt, M.C. and O'Dowd, K.J. (1985). Epidemiology of osteoporosis and osteoporotic fractures. *Epidemiol Rev.* **7:** 178–208.

Currie, A.L., Reid, D.M., Brown, N. and Nuki, G. (1986). An epidemiological study of fracture of the neck of femur. *Health Bull (Edin).* **44:** 143–148.

Delmi, M., Rapin, C.-H., Bengoa, J.-M., Delmas, P.D., Vasey, H. and Bonjour, J.-P. (1990). Dietary supplementation in elderly patients with fractured neck of the femur. *Lancet.* **335:** 1013–1016.

Eriksson, S.A.V. and Lindgren, J.U. (1989). Outcome of falls in women: endogenous factors associated with fracture. *Age Ageing.* **18:** 303–308.

Evans, J.G., Prudham, D. and Wandless, I. (1979). A prospective study of fractured proximal femur: incidence and outcome. *Public Health.* **93:** 235–241.

Evans, J.G., Wandless, I. and Prudham, D. (1980). A prospective study of fractured proximal femur; hospital differences. *Publ Hlth Lond.* **94:** 149–154.

Finsen, V. (1988). Improvements in general health among the elderly: a factor in the rising incidence of hip fractures? *J Epidemiol Community Health.* **42:** 200–203.

Greatorex, I.F. (1988). Proximal femoral fractures: an assessment of the outcome of health care in elderly people. *Community Medicine.* **10:** 203–210.

Hansson, L.I., Leder, L., Svensson, K. and Thorngren, K.-G. (1982). Incidence of fractures of the distal radius and proximal femur. *Acta Orthop Scand.* **53:** 721–726.

Harper, C.M. and Lyles, Y.M. (1988). Physiology and complications of bed rest. *J Am Geriatr Soc.* **36:** 1047–1054.

Heaney, R.P. (1990). Osteoporosis made easy (editorial). *J Am Geriatr Soc.* **38:** 1159–1160.

Hedlund, R., Ahlbom, A. and Lindgren, U. (1985). Hip fracture incidence in Stockholm 1972–1981. *Acta Orthop Scand.* **57:** 30–34.

Hedlund, R., Lindgren, U. and Ahlbom, A. (1987). Age- and sex-specific incidence of femoral neck and trochanteric fractures. An analysis based on 20,538 fractures in Stockholm County, Sweden 1972–1981. *Clin Orthop Rel Res.* **222:** 132–139.

Heidrich, F.E., Stergachis, A. and Gross, K.M. (1991). Diuretic drug use and the risk for hip fracture. *Ann Intern Med.* **115:** 1–6.

Hibbs, P.J. (1988). *Pressure area care for the City and Hackney Health Authority.*

HMSO (1989). *Hospital In-patient Enquiry: in-patient and day case trends 1979–1985.*

Holbrook, T.L., Barrett-Connor, E. and Wingard, D.L. (1988). Dietary calcium and risk of hip fracture: 14-year prospective population study. *Lancet.* **2:** 1046–1049.

Holmberg, S., Conradi, P., Kalen, R. and Thorngren, K.-G. (1986). Mortality after cervical hip fracture. 3002 patients followed for 6 years. *Acta Orthop Scand.* **57:** 8–11.

Jensen, J.S. and Bagger, J. (1982). Long term social prognosis after hip fractures. *Acta Orthop Scand.* **53:** 97–101.

Johnell, O., Nilsson, B.E. (1985). Hip fracture and accident disposition. *Acta Orthop Scand.* **56:** 302–304.

Katz, S., Heiple, K.G., Downs, T.D., Ford, A.B. and Scott, C.P. (1967). Long term course of 147 patients with fracture of the hip. *Surg Gyn Obstet.* **124:** 1219–1230.

Knowelden, J., Buhr, A.J. and Dunbar, O. (1964). Incidence of fractures in persons over 35 years of age. A report to the MRC Working Party on Fractures in the Elderly. **18:** 130–141.

Law, M.R., Wald, N.J. and Meade, T.W. (1991). Strategies for prevention of osteoporosis and hip fracture. *Br Med J.* **303:** 453–459.

Lawton, J.O., Baker, M.R. and Dickson, R.A. (1983). Femoral neck fractures – two populations. *Lancet.* **2:** 70–72.

Lewinnek, G.E., Kelsey, J., White, A.A. and Kreiger, N.J. (1980). The significance and a comparative analysis of the epidemiology of hip fractures. *Clin Orthop.* **152:** 35–43.

Lewis, A.F. (1981). Fracture of neck of the femur: changing incidence. *Br Med J.* **283:** 1217–1220.

Little, R.A. and Stoner, H.B. (1981). Body temperature after accidental injury. *Br J Surg.* **68:** 221–224.

Melton, L.J. III and Riggs, B.L. (1985). Risk factors for injury after a fall. *Clin Geriatr Med.* **1:** 525–36.

Melton, L.J. III and Riggs, B.L. (1987). Epidemiology of age-related fractures. In *The Osteoporotic Syndrome.* Alvioli, L.V. (ed.). New York: Grune and Stratton.

Miller, S.W.M. and Evans, J.G. (1985). Fractures of the distal forearm in Newcastle: an epidemiological survey. *Age Ageing.* **14:** 155–158.

Need, A.G., Nordin, B.E.C., Horowitz, M. and Morris, H.A. (1990). Osteoporosis. New insights from bone densitometry. *J Am Geriatr Soc.* **38:** 1153–1158.

Nevitt, M.C., Cummings, S.R., Kidd, S. and Black, D. (1989). Risk factors for recurrent non-syncopal falls. A prospective study. *JAMA.* **261:** 2663–2668.

Newton-John, H.F. and Morgan, D.B. (1968). Osteoporosis: disease or senescence? *Lancet.* **1:** 232–233.

Pryor, G.A., Williams, D.R.R., Myles, J.W. and Anand, J.K. (1988). Team management of the elderly patient with hip fracture. *Lancet.* **1:** 401–403.

Rashiq, S. and Logan, R.F.A. (1986). Role of drugs in fractures of the femoral neck. *Br Med J.* **292:** 861–863.

Ray, W.A., Griffin, M.R., Downey, W. and Melton, L.J. (1989). Long-term use of thiazide diuretics and risk of hip fracture. *Lancet.* **1:** 687–690.

Royal College of Physicians (1989). *Fractured Neck of Femur. Prevention and Management.* London, Royal College of Physicians of London.

Schapira, D. (1988). Physical exercise in the prevention and treatment of osteoporosis. *J Roy Soc Med.* **81:** 461–463.

Spector, T.D., Cooper, C. and Lewis, A.F. (1990). Trends in admissions for hip fracture in England and Wales, 1968–85. *Br Med J.* **300:** 1173–1174.

Speechley, M., Tinetti, M. (1991). Falls and injuries in frail and vigorous community elderly persons. *J Am Geriatr Soc.* **39:** 46–52.

Thomas, T.G. and Steven, R.S. (1974). Social effects of fractures of the neck of the femur. *Br Med J.* **3:** 456–458.

Wasnich, R.D., Benfante, R.J., Yano, K., Heilbrun, L. and Vogel, J.M. (1983). Thiazide effect on the mineral content of bone. *N Engl J Med.* **309:** 344–347.

Wickham, C.A.C., Walsh, K., Cooper, C., Barker, D.J.P., Margetts, B.M., Morris,

J. and Bruce, S.A. (1989). Dietary calcium, physical activity, and risk of hip fracture: a prospective study. *Br Med J.* **299**: 889–892.

Wong, P.C.N. (1966). Fracture epidemiology in a mixed south-eastern Asian community (Singapore). *Clin Orthop Rel Res.* **45:** 55–61.

Chapter 4 —————————

Balance, gait, and falling

Introduction

Falling at any age is the result of a complex interaction of factors with a common endpoint. A completed fall requires several elements; vulnerability, environmental hazard and exposure (Henker, 1987), or more simply, liability and opportunity. If there is no 'opportunity' to fall, for example if someone is lying on the floor, it does not matter how unstable they are (how 'liable' to fall), a fall will not occur. However, when walking along a tight-rope, a situation with a very large 'opportunity to fall', only someone with excellent balance, and therefore a very small 'liability to fall', would avoid falling. In young people, the opportunity element is generally more important. Falls in young people are commonly associated with more extreme movements stressing balance, and tend to occur in situations such as potentially hazardous leisure activities, or alternatively when liability has been increased because of alcohol. In the elderly, however, liability to fall seems to be dominant, and falls tend to occur with relatively minor degrees of stress on the balance mechanism.

For falls to occur during any activities at any age, postural control must be impaired relative to the amount by which it is stressed, and falls occurring during 'normal' activities suggest a greater impairment of postural control. The assumption that falls are the result of impaired control of gait and balance underlies the study of these factors in the elderly (both those who have fallen and those who have not) as an important part of studying falls generally.

Normal balance

The upright human body is basically unstable, with a very small support base relative to its height, and it becomes even more unstable on movement. A complicated neuromuscular system has developed to maintain this unstable position, remaining upright being an activity in which muscular corrections

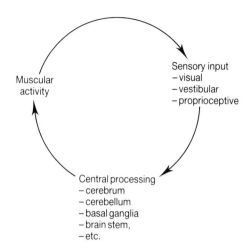

Fig. 4.1   Feedback loop controlling balance

are continually made on the basis of proprioceptive information about body position. Standing still is in fact anything but 'still'.

A complex feedback loop controls the system (Fig. 4.1). Information for the control centres in various parts of the brain comes from a number of important sensory inputs, which give the brain a picture of where the body and its constituent parts are in space. Vision is probably the most important of these, but information also comes from the vestibular apparatus in the inner ear and from various proprioceptors throughout the body. The proprioceptors provide information from muscle spindles, joints and skin surfaces, and the joints of the neck are particularly important. More information is provided than is necessary if all sensory inputs are working normally (i.e. there is redundancy of information), thus it is normally possible to remain upright and steady with the eyes closed or in the dark. Central processing occurs in many areas of the brain, including the cerebellum, the brainstem, the basal ganglia and the sensorimotor and association cortex, and the efferent limb is the outflow from the brain via spinal cord and peripheral nerves to limb and trunk muscles.

Assessment of the contributions of the various sensory and motor factors in maintenance of posture is not straightforward, mainly because if one element is impaired, the others can compensate to a greater or lesser degree. This means that interpreting problems with postural stability or predicting difficulties produced by sensory or motor damage is difficult.

The nervous system mechanisms responsible for motor control have components that are organised hierarchically. At the lowest level there is the spinal stretch reflex system with a latency of 40–50 msec. The next level is the long latency automatic postural response system (latency approximately 100 msec), with responses beginning in muscles closest to the base of support and spreading proximally in a stereotyped way. Finally, there are integrative mechanisms coordinating sensory inputs from vestibular, visual and somatosensory systems.

Age changes in the high level integrative mechanisms have been demonstrated. Cutaneous sensation and proprioception show increased thresholds for excitability with age. There is a reduction in spatial visual sensitivity, especially to low frequency spatial stimuli and slow moving targets, and this low frequency visual information is important for postural stabilisation. There is a reduction in vestibular function with ageing, which may interfere with the capacity of higher integrative processes within the central nervous system to deal with conflicting sensory information. In health the vestibular system appears to provides an internal orientational reference which is of critical importance in resolving conflict between different sources of sensory information during postural control.

There are very small changes in spinal stretch reflexes with age, leading to minor prolongation of latency, but these are probably of limited functional importance. There are, however, changes in long latency postural responses in the elderly compared to the young. There are increases in latency of distal muscles, disruption of the temporal sequencing of distal and proximal muscle activation, and increased variability in amplitude of contraction.

These age-related changes in adaptation and sensory organisation lead to marked deterioration in postural control in the elderly compared to the young when reduced or conflicting sensory information is provided, but the ability to adapt to these difficult sensory situations is retained to some extent (Woollacott et al., 1986). These findings would fit in with the tendency of the elderly to cope adequately with situations where stress on balance mechanisms is modest but to run into problems if balance is stressed to a greater extent.

Fine control of posture is immensely complex. Muscle activity (measured using electromyograms) in various postural muscles in response to unexpected displacements is extremely rapid, in some cases so fast that it starts before posture begins to be disturbed, so that it seems to anticipate the movement. Postural responses are also extremely sensitive, and have been shown to sense movement of approximately the diameter of a red blood cell (Marsden et al., 1981).

If balance is disturbed then various rescue mechanisms come into play to try to avoid loss of balance. To start with attempts are made by swaying to try to correct the initial derangement. If that is not sufficient, staggering (extending the area of support in the direction of the impending fall) and 'sweeping' movements (rapid movement of a limb to act as an inertia paddle) occur. If these rescue responses fail, then fall-breaking reactions are invoked, such as putting out the arms to break a fall. As well as making you more liable to fall, being old makes you more likely to land on the floor if you stumble, as these rescue and fall-breaking responses seem to be less efficient in the elderly.

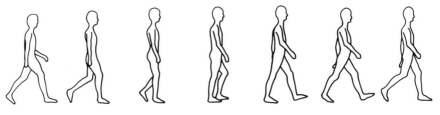

Fig. 4.2

Normal gait

Walking consists of repetitive, reciprocal movements, programmed as coordinated patterns involving the extremities and trunk, producing progressive motion (Fig. 4.2). There are two phases. The swing phase, during which the foot is lifted and swung forwards, and the stance phase when the foot is planted on the ground and moves backwards relative to the trunk, follow one another (Fig. 4.3). These sequential movements are caused by patterned ankle, knee and hip movements. There are also associated movements of other parts of the body, such as trunk, head and arms. The pattern generator is probably in the spinal cord (it certainly is in cats), and a spinal gait patterning mechanism is responsible for the automatic 'stepping' movements seen in newborn babies. Spinal cord activity is modulated by brainstem locomotor centres, basal ganglia, cerebellum, motor cortex and afferent input.

Normal and abnormal gaits are described in terms of the walking cycle. This is the time interval between successive floor contacts of one foot. During each walking cycle there are two periods of single limb support and two brief periods of double limb support (when one leg is about to begin the swing

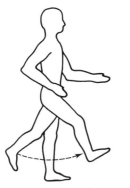
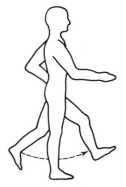

Right leg in swing phase.   Left leg in swing phase.
Left leg in stance phase   Right leg in stance phase

Fig. 4.3   Diagrams showing phases of gait (swing and stance)

phase and the other leg has just finished it). Variation in walking speeds is largely related to change in stride length rather than step frequency.

Assessment of balance and gait

The assessment of the control of posture and balance (and the contributions of the various elements which control them) has been carried out with relatively crude tools. Maintaining static posture involves complex neuromuscular interactions, but it's study has largely been via measurement of postural sway during quiet standing, perhaps analogous to studying cardiac function by measuring blood pressure alone.

Romberg observed in 1851 that subjects with tabes dorsalis swayed more on standing still than normals – the basis of the Romberg test – and since then attempts have been made to quantify this postural sway. In general the measurements have been made using equipment which produces a summation of all movements in one or more directions – an ataxiameter – or which produces a numerical or diagrammatic representation of the maximum sway in one or more directions (usually two directions at right angles) – an ataxiagraph. In each case it is fair to say that major simplifications are made in the analysis of the movement, since postural sway is a complex combination of movements in several planes and at several levels of the body. Measurements have been made of movements of head, waist, shoulders, or the position of centre of force measured at the feet. In some cases movements of two parts of the body have been measured simultaneously (e.g. head and hips, feet and waist), confirming that the body does not move rigidly during quiet standing but that different segments move in different ways and at different rates (Downton, 1990).

Measurement of gait has been somewhat more sophisticated, often using numerous simultaneous measurements of joint movements, positions of the feet, and muscle potentials. Temporal-spatial parameters (that is the basic timing and positional characteristics of gait) provide information about gait speed, step length (distance between consecutive foot falls) and stride length (distance between consecutive footfalls of the same foot) (Fig. 4.4). These can be measured at a simple level with stopwatch and tape measure, or complex electronic equipment can be used. However, simple recording of the time taken to walk a measured distance or a set number of steps may give sufficient information in a clinical setting.

Timing of the different phases of gait (swing time, single stance time, and double stance time) requires more complicated equipment, but foot placement characteristics, such as step and stride length, step width, foot angle and left–right symmetry, can be determined by observation and measurement of footprint patterns. (Fig. 4.4) These sorts of measurements are descriptions of motion independent of the forces which cause it, and are only partial descriptions without kinetic data, which describe the forces and moments

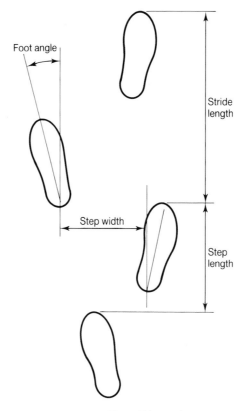

Fig. 4.4 The walking cycle

involved in motion. However, measurements of forces and moments increase the complexity of assessment, and except for specialised research, probably do not add much clinically useful information.

In clinical situations, much qualitative information about gait can be gained using the 'get-up and go test' (Mathias et al., 1986), during which the subject stands up from a chair, walks a short distance, turns around, returns, and sits down again. This test has recently been refined to allow quantification (Podsiadlo and Richardson, 1991). Other, similar 'performance oriented' mobility assessments have also been described (Tinetti, 1986).

Importance of various aspects of postural control

Vision

Of the three main sensory inputs upon which postural control depends (visual, vestibular and proprioceptive) the importance of vision has been most extensively studied. The almost universal finding that sway is greater with eyes closed than with eyes open demonstrates its importance.

Vision gives information about movement of head and body relative to surroundings and vice versa. It also tells us which direction is up – information deduced from such features as the horizon, walls of buildings, direction of bubbles rising in water or falling objects – and how our surroundings are oriented relative to 'up'. Visual information seems to be the most important input that the body considers when determining balance, to the extent that in situations of conflicting information, balance may in fact be lost when visual information is misleading. This has been shown in the 'hanging room' experiments, where misleading visual information overrides correct prop- rioceptive input (Lee and Lishman, 1975). Most people are familiar with the hallucination of movement that may be produced when sitting in a stationary train watching the moving train on the next platform, or the feeling of moving backwards when being passed by a faster train moving in the same direction. Sea sickness is thought to be related to the conflicting visual and vestibular information received on a moving boat, particularly when the horizon is not visible. The ability of visual information to override other sensory inputs about position and balance has been exploited for entertainment in optical illusions.

Vision seems to be particularly important when other sensory input is reduced or impaired, for example in amputees (Dornan et al., 1978). There may be an increase in visual dependence with increased age (Pyykko et al., 1990), though this has not always been shown, and it may be a result of peripheral nerve impairment in the very elderly, interfering with their proprioceptive input. However, women seem to be more 'field dependent' (that is they rely more on the spatial framework provided by vision) than men (Witkin et al., 1954), and it may be that, in conjunction with the tendency of women to have a narrower walking and standing base than men (Fig. 4.5), this is one factor in the higher frequency of falls in elderly women. Elderly fallers have been shown to have more errors in visual perception of verticality and horizontality than non-fallers (Tobis et al., 1981).

Vestibular function

The postural disturbance of someone with acute vestibular failure demons- trates the potential importance of vestibular function in maintenance of balance, but in fact the little evidence available suggests that vestibular deprivation is of secondary importance in the maintenance of posture. The vestibular apparatus, although an important part of the system which maintains balance, has another function, that of maintaining visual fixation. In order to make sure that the object of visual fixation is seen by the area of the retina with maximum resolution and best colour perception (the macula) the position of the eyes must be maintained despite movement of the head. Again, there is a feedback loop. Sensory input tells the central control areas

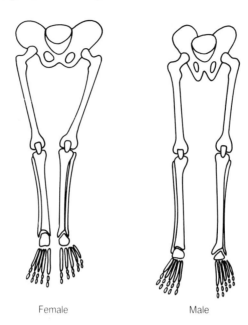

Female   Male

Fig. 4.5   Different stance positions of males and females because of configuration of pelvis

how posture and the visual field are changing in relation to the environment, and motor responses then maintain the stability of the body and direction of gaze.

The two aspects of the system are clearly interrelated but the importance of the various aspects differs depending on whether postural stability or visual fixation is seen as the primary aim. For simple postural control, the vestibular apparatus is less important than visual and somatosensory input. Thus individuals with bilateral damage to vestibular function can maintain balance quite adequately under normal circumstances. They do, however, run into problems when more complex positional information has to be processed, such as walking on uneven ground, or when other sensory inputs are reduced, such as in the dark.

The way in which the vestibular apparatus works is poorly understood, partly because of the difficulties of obtaining suitable specimens, both in health and disease, of an organ which is entirely contained within the temporal bone. Preparation artefacts have confused those studying the anatomy and pathology, and the ability of other systems to compensate for vestibular damage have confused the physiologist and pathophysiologist. It is known, however, that the semicircular canals sense movement because of the inertia of their various solid and liquid components. Since the three canals in one ear are at right angles to each other they can sense movement in any direction, and the complementary position of the canals in the other ear means that complex angular acceleration and deceleration can be analysed.

Abnormalities of vestibular function, measured using a tipping table, have been found significantly more commonly with increasing age, but there does not appear to be any correlation between this age-related vestibular dysfunction and sway (Brocklehurst et al., 1982). Sway in those with vestibular disease, however, has been shown to be greater in elderly than in young subjects (Norre et al., 1987).Vestibular abnormalities (usually demonstrated by means of opticokinetic nystagmus and caloric testing) have been shown to be associated with, and therefore perhaps a cause of dizziness (Drachmann and Hart, 1972) but their relationship to falls is not clear.

Although hearing would not intuitively seem to be one of the important sensory inputs for maintaining balance, significantly greater sway has been reported in subjects with noise-induced hearing loss compared with controls (Juntunen et al., 1987; Era and Heikkinen, 1985) and sway correlated with the degree of hearing impairment. This may demonstrate subclinical disturbance of the vestibular system amongst subjects with noise-induced hearing loss. Vestibular function is discussed further in Chapter 6.

Proprioception

Somatosensory input is often underestimated as an element of normal and defective postural control. Vital information about the position of the body in space and the relative positions of various body parts is constantly being transmitted by muscle and joint proprioceptors, especially those in the lower limbs and the neck.

Proprioceptors in the cervical spine joints are particularly important, but information from all the 'postural' muscles also contributes, as does information from skin touch receptors. Cervical spine mechanoreceptors contribute significantly to static postural sensation and to the awareness of head and neck movement (Wyke, 1979). Local anaesthetic infiltration of the cervical apophyseal joints in normal volunteers produces subjective feelings of unsteadiness whilst standing and walking (de Jong et al., 1977), and people with cervical spine disorders often complain of similar symptoms.

Amputees (who have lost some of their proprioceptive input) sway more than normals, though they are able to compensate to some extent with vision (Fernie and Holliday, 1978). Mechanical vibration of the calf muscles, which disturbs somatic proprioception, also increases postural sway (Eklund and Lofstedt, 1970), though again the effect of this is most obvious in the absence of visual input. Muscle spindle proprioceptive sensitivity is poorer in very old subjects than in younger age groups, and disruption of proprioception has a greater effect in the very elderly than in younger subjects (Pyykko et al., 1990).

Central control of posture

The importance of central control areas in the maintenance of balance is largely demonstrated by the results of pathology in those areas. A single lesion, or lesions in a single site, can produce gait and balance problems (e.g. Parkinsons disease, cerebellar ataxia) or multiple lesions may be required (e.g. gait apraxia produced by multiple cortical or subcortical infarcts). Because of brain plasticity and the ability of other areas to compensate for damage, the effects of an individual lesion are difficult to predict. For both posture and gait, the measurable difference from normal is the effect of what remains after the system has compensated for an abnormality as far as it is able; it is not a measure of the abnormality itself. Therefore the same measured abnormality in different subjects may be the result of quite different pathologies. However, damage to any of the areas of the central nervous system impinging on balance and gait, or to connections to or from those areas, may produce instability.

Changes in postural control with age

As mentioned above, standing still consists of continuous movement correcting balance (Fig. 4.6). In various studies, the postural control of children has

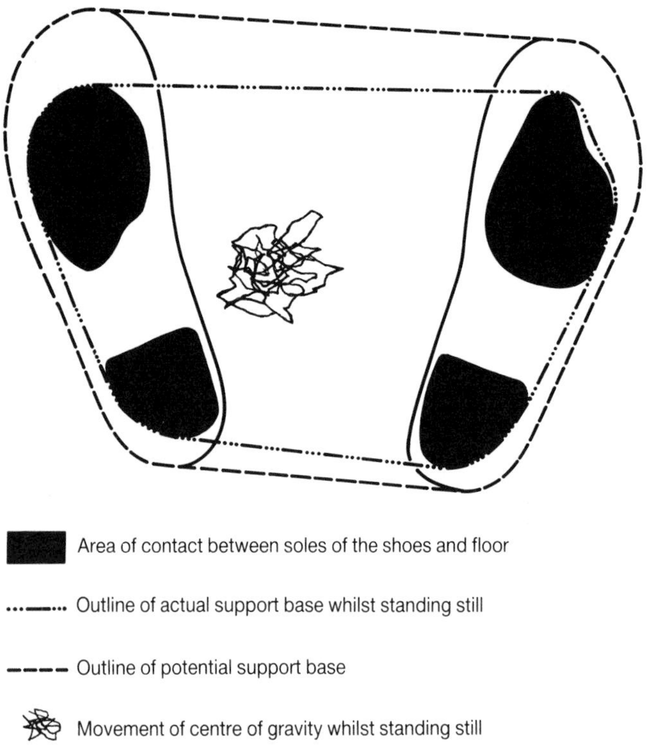
Area of contact between soles of the shoes and floor
Outline of actual support base whilst standing still
Outline of potential support base
Movement of centre of gravity whilst standing still

Fig. 4.6 Movement of the centre of gravity whilst standing 'still' demonstrated by force plate measurements of static balance

been measured and found to be less than that of adults. As children mature, their balance improves. The effect of increasing age on sway was first demonstrated in 1939, when Hellebrandt and Braun (1939) measured the postural sway of 111 subjects aged between 3 and 86 years. They found that there was a 'tendency for the young and the old to be less stable than the young adult and the middle-aged subject'.

Sheldon (1963) also looked at postural sway in a wide age range (6–97 years) of subjects and seems to have been the first to consider that measurement of postural sway might be useful to study the liability of the elderly to fall. He tested two different positions of stance: both standing with the feet comfortably apart, the first with the eyes shut and the second with the subject looking directly at the pencil registering his or her movements, trying to keep it as still as possible for one minute. This test demonstrated that young and middle-aged adults were able to control their sway more accurately than either children or the elderly. Interestingly, approximately a third of subjects over 60 years appeared to be unable to control their sway in response to this visual feedback.

Hasselkus and Shambes (1975) also observed the effect of age on sway, taking two experimental groups, aged 21–30 years and 73–80 years ('female volunteers who had no known neurological or severe physiological disorders'). Sway was significantly greater in the elderly group than the young group. Intra-individual variation was great in both groups but inter-individual variation was greater in the elderly. Studies of sway in exclusively elderly groups has not, however, always shown a clear relationship between increasing age and deteriorating postural control, particularly in those studies which have examined representative community elderly populations (Downton et al., 1991).

In summary, the elderly sway more on average when standing still than do young and middle-aged adults. However, as with many factors that change with age, variability increases (that is, the normal range becomes wider) with increasing age, and there is overlap between the 'normal ranges' for younger adults and those for the elderly.

The way in which the elderly stand is different from posture at younger ages (Fig. 4.7). There is a greater tendency to stoop, partly because of the development of a dorsal kyphosis, though this is not universal. The head tends to be thrown forward, and there is often a degree of flexion at the hips, knees and ankles. Although it is sometimes suggested that such a posture is adopted because of balance difficulties, there is no evidence to support this (Cunha et al., 1987).

Changes in gait with age

The gait of the elderly has been quite extensively studied. Healthy elderly men show significantly slower walking speed, shorter stride length, greater

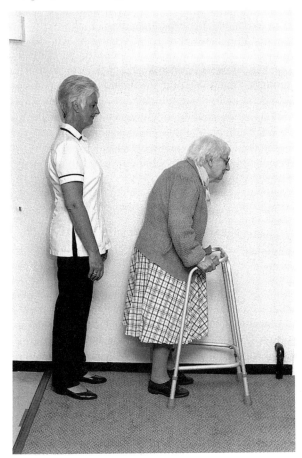

Fig. 4.7 Posture in young and old subjects

degrees of out-toeing, and longer time spent in stance with shorter time in swing phases than young men. This results in longer walking cycle duration. In addition there is slightly greater stride width, less hip rotation and knee flexion during swing phase and less ankle extension at the end of stance phase. Vertical movements of the head are less. There is however, no change in rhythmicity or reproducibility of successive stride dimensions and temporal components of gait. '[The] walking performance of the older men gave the impression of a guarded or restrained type of walking in an attempt to obtain maximum stability and security' (Murray et al., 1969). Walking speed declines significantly with age, though the decline is small, being less than 1 per cent per year (Bendall et al., 1989).

Elderly women demonstrate similar changes, with shorter step length, larger number of steps per minute, slower gait speed and reduced swing to support ratio. In addition, elderly women have higher body centre of gravity to height ratios than young women (Finley et al., 1969). They also demonstrate increased muscle activity on walking, suggesting that this kind of 'safer' walking may be more energy 'expensive', with reduction in kinetic efficiency (Guimaraes and Isaacs, 1980). These age changes are much less apparent if subjects are highly selected to exclude pathology (Gabell and Nayak, 1984) and are more apparent in unselected elderly (Imms and Edholm, 1981).

There are two elements of gait – balance control and gait patterning. The first includes stride width and double support time and the second includes step length and stride time. An increase in stride width and double support time (balance control elements) leads to greater stability and/or compensation for instability, and an increase in the variability of these elements is likely to lead to greater instability. An increase in variability of step length and stride time (gait patterning elements) implies failure of gait patterning and may predispose to falls. A study of healthy elderly and young subjects showed little variability in gait patterning parameters, but higher variability for balance related parameters in both age groups. There was little difference between the two age groups in either gait patterning or balance related parameters. This suggests either that gait patterning is more consistent at all ages, or that balance mechanisms are better able to cope with considerable variations, implying substantial adaptive power within the balance control system (Gabell and Nayak, 1984). The lack of difference between healthy elderly and young subjects suggests that impaired gait and balance in the elderly are due to pathology rather than physiological age changes.

There is a relationship between gait parameters, habitual levels of activity, and mobility in a more general sense (ability to get up from a chair, negotiate steps, etc.) (Bendall et al., 1989). Those who are less mobile and active have more marked 'age-related' gait changes than those who maintain activity (Ring et al., 1988). Although in the absence of a longitudinal study it is difficult to prove which came first, it is quite likely that reduction in activity levels leads to secondary gait and balance changes.

Normal gait depends on normal function, not only of the neuromuscular system, but also of the skeletal, circulatory and respiratory systems, in a highly coordinated and integrated manner. Injury or disease in any of these systems can lead to impaired gait, and the differential diagnosis of abnormal gait is very wide.

Relevance of abnormalities of postural control to falls and falling

What is the relationship between impaired gait and balance and falls in the elderly? Although studies have shown relationships between 'poor balance' and falls, it is not clear which is cause and which is effect (did the poor balance cause the fall or vice versa?). Measurement of balance in 'fallers' occurs after the fall, so that an effect of the fall on balance cannot be excluded.

Subjective postural disturbances are common in the elderly. Postural control as measured by sway seems to be impaired in the elderly, particularly in those with pathological changes of various kinds. There is also evidence that 'impaired' subjects sway more than non-impaired. This has been shown for vision (Stevens and Tomlinson, 1971), hearing (Juntunen et al., 1987), vestibular function (Norre and Forrez, 1986), muscle proprioception (Eklund and Lofstedt, 1970) and joint proprioception (de Jong et al., 1977). Sway has been shown to be greater in demented subjects (Visser, 1983), which may indicate problems with central processing. The increase in sway with age found in many studies may therefore be related to an accumulation of pathology. Impaired postural control is common amongst elderly patients in hospital (Ring et al., 1988).

This impaired postural control in elderly subjects seems to be associated with an increased likelihood of falling. An association between sway and a history of falls in the previous 12 months has been shown in institutionalised elderly subjects, but the differences between the groups were small, and there was a large overlap between fallers and non-fallers (Fernie et al., 1982). Several other studies using various non-randomly selected groups of elderly have shown statistically significant, but small, differences in some measurements of sway in subgroups of elderly fallers, but measurements of balance in a representative group of community living elderly did not show a significant difference in sway between fallers and non-fallers (Downton et al., 1991).

A relationship between increased sway and falls was first noted by Sheldon in 1963. His subject group included some elderly living at home and some in longstay wards. He found a subgroup who were unable to control their sway in response to a visual feedback, and commented that 'the majority [of that subgroup] had actually sustained one or more falls'. It is interesting that the differences between his controls and his elderly subjects were much more marked in the direct vision test (where subjects attempted to minimise their sway with a visual feedback) than the eyes closed test.

Because falls and balance disturbances are common in the elderly, and sway increases with age and impairment, it is assumed that the two factors are causally related. However, the closeness of this assumed relationship between symptomatic balance disorders and objective measurements of balance is uncertain, and the direction of causation is not known. The evidence is limited, inconclusive, and often contradictory. The complexity of the physiological mechanisms which control balance, and the vast number of factors that are associated with clinical 'balance disorders' means that this uncertainty and imprecision should not be surprising. In addition, many of the factors which in the elderly could be said to produce a 'liability' to fall will not cause a fall unless an 'opportunity' to fall is also present. Falls can occur at any age, but the relative contributions of 'liability' and 'opportunity' seem to differ at different ages, and at different times in an individual. Even in the elderly a proportion of falls are due to simple trips or slips, such as can occur at any age. Abnormalities of the balance control mechanisms (which might theoretically be detected by balance measurements) will only impinge on the 'liability' to fall and are probably unconnected to the 'opportunity' to fall.

Balance measurements do not distinguish reliably between those with and without symptomatic balance disorders. They cannot predict which subjects will fall and at present are too imprecise to give clues as to where any defect in balance maintenance may lie. There is little information about the role of intervention in those with 'poor' balance, though postural sway biofeedback has been used to reestablish stance stability in hemiplegic patients (Shumway-Cook et al., 1988). In order for balance assessment to be useful there has to be a much clearer delineation of the physiological and pathological status of those whose balance is measured, so that correlations between measurements and pathophysiology can be determined. Static balance may not be a particularly useful parameter to measure, and effort might be better expended on the study of dynamic balance, either in the study of gait or using tests that stress static balance. Although these areas are more complex and more difficult to quantify, it seems likely that they bear a closer relationship to clinical balance disorders (Wolfson et al., 1986).

In clinical practice, simple assessments of posture and gait can provide much useful information about functional balance. The observation of balance during quiet standing, a Romberg test, the response to a minor balance stress (for example, a gentle push on the chest) and a simple mobility assessment (such as the 'get up and go' test) can highlight areas of impairment and will almost certainly pick up those elderly with significant balance problems.

References

Bendall, M.J., Bassey, E.J. and Pearson, M.B. (1989). Factors affecting walking speed of elderly people. *Age Ageing*. **18:** 327–332.
Brocklehurst, J.C., Robertson, D. and James-Groom, P. (1982). Clinical correlates of sway in old age – sensory modalities. *Age Ageing*. **11:** 1–10.
Cunha, U., Leduc, M., Nayak, U.S.L. and Isaacs, B. (1987). Why do old people stoop? *Arch Gerontol Geriatr*. **6:** 363–369.
de Jong, P.T.V.M., de Jong, J.M.B.V., Cohen, B. and Jongkees, L.B.W. (1977). Ataxia and nystagmus induced by injection of local anaesthetics in the neck. *Ann Neurol*. **1:** 240–246.
Dornan, J., Fernie, G.R. and Holliday, P.J. (1978). Visual input: its importance in the control of postural sway. *Arch Phys Med Rehabil*. **59:** 586–591.
Downton, J.H. (1990). The clinical relevance of balance assessment in the elderly – a personal review. *Clin Rehab*. **4:** 305–312.
Downton, J.H., Sayegh, A. and Andrews, K. (1991). Preliminary study of measurements of sway in an elderly community population. *Clin Rehab*. **5:** 187–194.
Drachmann, D.A. and Hart, C.W. (1972). An approach to the dizzy patient. *Neurology*. **22:** 323–334.
Eklund, G. and Lofstedt, L. (1970). Biomechanical analysis of balance. *Biomed Eng*. **5:** 333–337.
Era, P. and Heikkinen, E. (1985). Postural sway during standing and unexpected

disturbance of balance in random samples of men of different ages. *J Gerontol.* **40:** 287–295.

Fernie, G.R., Gryfe, C.I., Holliday, P.J. and Llewellyn, A. (1982). The relationship of postural sway in standing to the incidence of falls in geriatric subjects. *Age Ageing.* **11:** 11–16.

Fernie, G.R. and Holliday, P.J. (1978). Postural sway in amputees and normal subjects. *J Bone Joint Surg.* **60A:** 895–898.

Finley, F.R., Cody, K.A. and Finizie, R.A. (1969). Locomotion patterns in elderly women. *Arch Phys Med Rehabil.* **50:** 140–146.

Gabell, A. and Nayak, U.S.L. (1984). The effect of age on variability of gait. *J Gerontol.* **39:** 662–666.

Guimaraes, R.M. and Isaacs, B. (1980). Characteristics of the gait in old people who fall. *Int Rehabil Med.* **2:** 177–180.

Hasselkus, B.R. and Shambes, G.M. (1975). Aging and postural sway in women. *J Gerontol.* **30:** 661–667.

Hellebrandt, F.A. and Braun, G.L. (1939). The influence of sex and age on the postural sway of man. *Am J Phys Anthropol.* **24:** 347–360.

Henker, F.O. (1987). Accident proneness and how to prevent it. *Clin Orthop.* **222:** 30–34.

Imms, F.J. and Edholm, O.G. (1981). Studies of gait and mobility in the elderly. *Age Ageing.* **10:** 147–156.

Juntunen, J., Matikainen, E., Ylikoski, J., Ylikoski, M., Ojala, M. and Vaheri, E. (1987). Postural body sway and exposure to high-energy impulse noise. *Lancet.* **2:** 261–264.

Lee, D.N. and Lishman, J.R. (1975). Visual proprioceptive control of stance. *J Hum Move Stud.* **1:** 87–95.

Marsden, C.D., Merton, P.A. and Morton, H.B. (1981). Human postural responses. *Brain.* **104:** 513–534.

Mathias, S., Nayak, U.S.L. and Isaacs, B. (1986). Balance in elderly patients: the 'get up and go' test. *Arch Phys Med Rehabil.* **67:** 387–9.

Murray, M.P., Kory, R.C. and Clarkson, B.H. (1969). Walking patterns in healthy old men. *J Gerontol.* **24:** 169–178.

Norre, M.E. and Forrez, G. (1986). Posture testing (posturography) in the diagnosis of peripheral vestibular pathology. *Arch Otorhinolaryngol.* **243:** 186–189.

Norre, M.E., Forrez, G. and Beckers, A. (1987). Posturography measuring instability in vestibular dysfunction in the elderly. *Age Ageing.* **16:** 89–93.

Peacock, M. (1985). Can fractures be prevented? In: Isaacs, B. (ed.) *Recent Advances in Geriatric Medicine 3.* pp. 177–191, Churchill Livingstone, Edinburgh.

Podsiadlo, D. and Richardson, S. (1991). The timed 'up and go': a test of basic functional mobility for frail elderly persons. *J Am Geriatr Soc.* **39:** 142–148.

Pyykko, I., Jantti, P. and Aalto, H. (1990). Postural control in elderly subjects. *Age Ageing.* **19:** 215–221.

Ring, C., Nayak, U.S.L. and Isaacs, B. (1988). Balance function in elderly people who have and who have not fallen. *Arch Phys Med Rehabil.* **69:** 261–264.

Sheldon, J.H. (1963). The effect of age on the control of sway. *Gerontol Clin.* **5:** 129–138.

Shumway-Cook, A., Anson, D. and Haller, S. (1988). Postural sway biofeedback: its effect on reestablishing stance stability in hemiplegic patients. *Arch Phys Med Rehabil.* **69:** 395–400.

Stevens, D.L. and Tomlinson, G.E. (1971). Measurement of human postural sway. *Proc Roy Soc Med.* **64:** 653–655.

Tinetti, M.E. (1986). Performance-oriented assessment of mobility problems in elderly patients. *J Am Geriatr Soc.* **34:** 119–126.

Tobis, J.S., Nayak, U.S.L. and Hoehler, F. (1981). Visual perception of verticality and horizontality among elderly fallers. *Arch Phys Med Rehabil.* **62:** 619–622.

Visser, H. (1983). Gait and balance in senile dementia of Alzheimer's type. *Age Ageing.* **12:** 296–301.

Witkin, H.A., Lewis, H.B., Herzman, M., Machover, K., Meissner, P., Bretnall, P. and Wapner, S. (1954). *Personality through perception: an experimental and clinical study.* New York, Harper.

Wolfson, L.I., Whipple, R., Amerman, P. and Kleinberg, A. (1986). Stressing the postural response. A quantitative method for testing balance. *J Am Geriatr Soc.* **34:** 845–850.

Woollacott, M.H., Shumway-Cook, A. and Nashner, L.M. (1986). Aging and posture control: changes in sensory organization and muscular coordination. *Int J Aging Hum Dev.* **23:** 97–114.

Wyke, B. (1979). Cervical articular contributions to posture and gait: their relation to senile disequilibrium. *Age Ageing.* **8:** 251–258.

Chapter 5 _____

Why do old people fall?

There are probably almost as many reasons why the elderly fall as there are elderly fallers. The potential causes of falls cover virtually the whole of clinical medicine, and also include physiological age changes, environmental causes and interactions between internal and external factors. Many of the diseases to which the elderly are prone increase risk of falling, and age-related changes in body systems often mean that an illness presents with, or leads to falling.

Changes with ageing and their relevance to falling

The elderly are in many ways different from the young, and it is possible to describe a number of characteristics of structure and function of elderly individuals which are recognised to be unlike those in younger people, though there is dispute about whether they are 'normal' findings or caused by disease states. Some of these differences have effects which impinge on balance and liability to fall, and to some extent may explain the greater tendency of old people to be unsteady and to fall in a variety of situations. Ageing of the various elements involved in maintenance of balance (see Chapter 4) could theoretically account for increasing instability with age.

Neurological changes

Describing and quantifying the neurological changes that occur with ageing is difficult. Structural and functional changes found in elderly individuals, but absent in younger ones, may be the result of physiological or pathological events. However, there is such wide variability in structural and functional changes found in ageing individuals that it is impossible to say that, in the absence of disease, there is any inevitable change with ageing. The vast majority of studies of neurological changes with ageing are cross-sectional rather than longitudinal, so that they may in fact be demonstrating a cohort effect rather than true age difference. Another difficulty with cross-sectional studies of age-related neurological changes is to obtain subjects without superimposed disease, as the prevalence of neurological disorders increases with increasing age, with some kind of neurological problem present in almost half of those of 75 and over (Broe et al., 1976). There is also little information about correlations between structural and functional changes, though a few studies have looked at the relationship between the two. For example, the number of plaques and neurofibrillary tangles found in brain tissue at autopsy has been shown to correlate with measures of cognitive function before death in subjects with dementia (Blessed et al., 1968).

There is no doubt that there are definite structural changes in the central nervous system in the elderly, such as reduced cell counts, increase in connective tissue, accumulation of lipofuscin, and so on. There is also some evidence of decrease in nerve conduction rate with age (Dorfman and Bosley, 1979). It has been suggested, however, that maintenance of reaction time (demonstrating speed of nerve conduction) depends on frequency of use rather than age. Reaction times for systems that are in constant use, such as muscles controlling speech, show much smaller changes with age than systems where use tends to decline with age, such as muscles controlling limb movements, suggesting that the decrease in reaction time is a form of 'disuse atrophy' (Nebes, 1978).

Certain 'abnormal' neurological findings (atrophy of the hand muscles, flexed posture, disorders of gait, static tremors, loss of vibration sense and tendon jerks in the lower limbs, and irregular, sluggish pupils) have been reported to be attributable to age rather than to current disease (Prakash and Stern, 1973), but since these abnormalities were found in admissions to a geriatric unit, the subjects were by definition not healthy. The reported loss of ankle jerks with age may be related to technique of examination rather than true loss of reflexes (Impallomeni et al., 1984).

The most consistent finding in studies of the neurological changes with age is loss of vibration sensation in the lower limbs. However, vibration is not a specific modality carried in a specific pathway. It probably travels in both dorsal columns and spinothalamic pathways and is appreciated bilaterally at thalamic level, and the relationship to proprioception is not clear. Assessment of proprioception is not easy, especially in the elderly, and reported findings are contradictory. Overall there does not seem to be a consistent association between impairment of proprioception and impaired vibration sensation in elderly subjects (MacLennan et al., 1980), nor does impaired proprioception appear to be related to age or to a history of falling (Brocklehurst et al., 1982). Increasing age, absent ankle jerks and impaired vibration sensation are, however, related in elderly subjects, suggesting that vibration changes may be due to peripheral nerve degeneration rather than posterior column damage (MacLennan et al., 1980).

Carefully carried out studies of neurological changes with ageing (consider-ing as far as possible those without neurological disease) have shown little consistent impairment of functioning, and have suggested that what changes are present may be caused by types of disuse atrophy (DeVries et al., 1985). Attempting to ascribe the liability of old people to fall to the neurological changes found with ageing is an attractive idea but the evidence available suggests that neurological diseases rather than 'physiological' age changes are responsible for the tendency to fall experienced by the elderly.

Ageing of the eye

Many of the features of the elderly eye represent physiological age changes in that they occur universally with ageing. The lens progressively increases in thickness throughout life, as a consequence becoming less flexible. Near vision becomes more difficult (presbyopia). In addition, the lens yellows and becomes relatively opacified, reducing the amount of light transmitted. The pupil becomes progressively smaller, though ability to constrict in response to light is retained. Dark adaptation deteriorates with age, partly because of the pupillary and lens changes, but also because of retinal changes. This is of particular importance as it significantly impairs vision where light intensity is low.

Cross-sectional studies show a decline in visual acuity with age, though longitudinal studies suggest that the decline is not uniform, and is partly accounted for by development of cataract, and to a lesser degree by other eye diseases (Milne, 1979). Thus the development of pathological changes in the eyes is a more important cause of the deterioration in vision with age than age-related physiological changes. The common causes of visual disability become much commoner with increasing age: cataract, glaucoma and senile macular degeneration all result in important functional visual problems for those elderly affected. In addition, cerebrovascular disease may cause visual field deficits, and diabetic and hypertensive vascular disease take their toll on the eyes of a proportion of the elderly.

Self-reported visual difficulties increase significantly with age (Gerson et al., 1989). However, assessments made by subjects themselves of visual change over five years do not necessarily agree with objective measurements (Milne, 1979), so relying on the elderly to judge for themselves when their vision has deteriorated is an unreliable method to identify potential problems. Some form of screening is needed.

Vestibular ageing

One of the problems associated with determining the effects of age on the vestibular apparatus is that there is a substantial ability within the system to compensate for damage to or deterioration of vestibular function. However, this ability to overcome vestibular dysfunction deteriorates with age, though vision can make up for this to some extent (Norre et al., 1987). In addition, the situation of the vestibular apparatus within the petrous temporal bone means that its anatomical study in health and disease is difficult.

There do appear to be histological changes in the vestibular primary afferent neurons and hair cells with age, and these seem to be confirmed by changes in conventional vestibular function tests (Oosterveld, 1983). This does not, however, mean that all symptoms of dizziness are caused by vestibular dysfunction. Although dizziness is a common complaint amongst elderly people, the causes of such symptoms are legion, and vestibular disorders alone account for a minority of such complaints (see Chapter 6).

Changes in gait and postural control with age

These are discussed in more detail in Chapter 4. There seems little doubt that postural control is impaired with increasing age, though the causes for this are probably 'pathological' rather than 'physiological'. The deterioration in ability to maintain static position should not necessarily increase the liability to fall until sway reaches such a degree that the centre of gravity comes to lie outside the margins of the base of support, and even then balance could be maintained if corrective postural responses were sufficient to counteract the sway. In fact, few falls occur whilst standing still (with the exception of some clearly defined pathological problems, such as loss of consciousness or postural hypotension), and the relevance of static postural control to falls is unclear.

The deterioration in postural control that has been demonstrated with increasing age is a marker of failure of compensatory mechanisms, and is part of the general loss of functional reserve that typifies ageing. Ability to respond to stress is reduced although function remains adequate in unstressed situations. The failure of compensatory balance mechanisms perhaps follows from slowing of messages within the feedback loop controlling balance. In the time taken for the message to reach central control areas from propriocep-tors, the displacing movement has continued and extended further than if transmission were faster. Because messages to postural muscles are also slower, the amount of movement required to control position can be estimated less accurately, producing the possibility of over- or under-correction and further loss of balance. This slowing of reaction times may be a function of generally reduced activity rather than an age change per se (Spirduso, 1975).

Because, during active motion, the centre of gravity moves outside the area of support frequently and to a much greater extent than whilst standing still, the potential for unbalanced movements and inaccurate corrections is grea-ter. Thus falls much more frequently occur during activity. The ability to correct unbalanced movements does seem to be impaired in the elderly, particularly the frail elderly who have had falls, and synergistic muscle actions to correct displacements seem to be incomplete and delayed in the elderly compared to young controls (Wolfson et al., 1986). The differences between age groups in postural sway are much more dramatic when sway in response to displacement of the centre of gravity is measured (Maki et al., 1990).

The frequency with which peripheral nerve problems are found in elderly subjects means that many elderly have impairment in the proprioceptive input to balance control feedback loops and therefore have to rely on vision rather than stretch reflexes (mediated through peripheral nerves) to maintain balance. Visual responses are substantially slower than stretch reflexes (150 ms vs 100 ms) and this therefore increases the latency with which disturbances of balance are sensed. In addition, the stretch reflex is involved in acute control of a sudden fall, and malfunction of this response in the elderly may explain why balance cannot so easily be regained when disturbed as in younger people.

The alterations in gait in the elderly described in Chapter 4 should again not of themselves result in increased liability to fall, and to some extent seem designed to improve stability. However, the reduction in hip rotation and knee flexion during swing phase result in the foot being lifted less during swing phase, and may account for the greater tendency of the elderly to trip. In the absence of pathology these changes probably do not have much effect on risk of falling, though the overall changes may lead to significant problems coping with some aspects of modern life, such as crossing roads using timed pedestrian crossings (Nelson et al., 1991). Stumbling, which may result from these gait changes, is a risk factor for later falls (Teno et al., 1990).

Gait assessment of elderly fallers compared to normal controls does show significant differences in many aspects of gait (Wolfson et al., 1990). 'Idiopathic gait disorder of the elderly', with consistent gait changes not explicable by disease states, appears to be a clinical entity (Hogan et al., 1987). However, it may not in fact increase likelihood of falling as about half of a gait disordered group, mean age 80 years, had a history of falls – approximately what would be expected for an unselected group of this age. Many elderly subjects with abnormal gaits have underlying pathological causes (Sudarsky and Ronthal, 1983) and potential causes of gait disorders include metabolic, cardiovascular and other disorders as well as neurological ones.

Autonomic dysfunction and postural hypotension

Autonomic dysfunction is more common in the elderly than in young subjects (Smith and Fasler, 1983), and is particularly manifest as postural hypotension, though not all postural hypotension is due to autonomic neuropathy. Little is known about age changes in the autonomic nervous system, but some degree of autonomic denervation does seem to occur with increasing age in healthy individuals (Collins et al., 1980).

Maintenance of blood pressure on standing depends on effective functioning of baroreceptors, the brainstem vasomotor centre, and myocardium and blood vessels, and disease in these areas can result in postural hypotension.

Neurological disease is well recognised to be associated with postural hypotension, particularly in those with autonomic neuropathies, Parkinson's disease and Shy–Drager syndrome, but it also occurs in those with cerebral infarcts, diffuse atherosclerosis, and spinal cord lesions. There also seem to be age-related changes apart from autonomic degeneration which lead to a higher risk of postural hypotension, in that postural hypotension may be present without other evidence of autonomic dysfunction. This may be related to atherosclerotic loss of distensibility of large vessels (Robinson et al., 1983).

Substantial numbers of elderly people have a significant drop in blood pressure on standing. Approximately 20 per cent of those over 65 have an orthostatic drop in blood pressure of 20 mmHg or more (Caird et al., 1973). The mechanism of this drop is not clear and is probably multifactorial. Potential factors include reduced baroreceptor sensitivity (Gribbin et al., 1971), excessive venous pooling (Caird et al., 1973), and autonomic dysfunction. The elderly are also more prone to postprandial hypotension (Lipsitz et al., 1983). Old people with impaired baroreceptor reflexes may have failure of cerebral autoregulation (Wollner et al., 1979) increasing the likelihood of symptoms if their blood pressure drops.

Not all those with a measured drop in blood pressure on standing have symptoms of postural dizziness, and not all those with postural dizziness have a measured drop in blood pressure on standing. Presumably those with a drop in blood pressure but no symptoms have more efficient cerebral autoregulation. It is possible that the presence of symptoms of cerebral hypoperfusion in association with orthostatic hypotension is also related to general health, hydration, and nutrition, and to intercurrent illnesses.

The relationship between postural hypotension and falling seems logical but is difficult to prove unless ambulatory blood pressure monitoring is in progress at the time of the fall. Demonstration of a drop in blood pressure on standing in someone who has fallen, particularly if associated with symptoms of dizziness or light-headedness, is assumed to show cause and effect, but this cannot be more than an assumption unless the hypotension is of such a degree as to produce loss of consciousness. Where evidence of autonomic dysfunction has been sought (for example using heart rate response to tilting) there has been no significant difference between healthy controls and fallers with many medical and neurological problems (Kirshen et al., 1984).

Case report

A 69 year-old man was referred to hospital as an emergency because of recurrent faints on the day of admission. He had previously been well and had no other symptoms. The only abnormal finding on examination was marked postural hypotension. The admitting doctor was puzzled, and speculated about various rare neurological syndromes associated with postural hypotension. The puzzle was solved two hours after admission when the patient passed a large melaena stool.

Musculoskeletal ageing

Total muscle mass declines with age, though again most studies are cross-sectional, and cohort effects of nutrition and lifestyle may be important. The decline in muscle mass is greater in men than women, and is due to a reduction in the number of muscle fibres. There is a reduction in maximal oxygen uptake with age, but this is largely because of cardiovascular changes (reduction in maximal heart rate, impaired myocardial contractility, increased stiffness of larger vessels) rather than any direct muscle changes. The muscle changes that are found are at least partly related to change in activity levels at different ages. Muscles which remain physically active, such as the diaphragm and vocal muscles, show much less change with age, and active elderly show better motor performance than inactive elderly (Rickli and Busch, 1986). Training can improve muscle strength even in nonagenarians (Fiatarone et al., 1990). Although changes in muscle strength are related more to levels of activity than age itself, many elderly have a degree of muscle weakness, particularly in the lower limbs, sufficient to have a significant effect on stability and walking, and lower limb muscle weakness has been identified as an important risk factor for falls (Whipple et al., 1987).

Osteoarthritis is so common that it can be considered as an age-related, almost 'physiological' event. Ageing of cartilage results in cells becoming less numerous, metabolic activities of cartilage cells declining, and a gradual decrease in the water content of cartilage. These changes result in a deterioration of the strength and elasticity of the cartilage, eventually leading to fibrillation and loss of cartilage from joint surfaces. This is followed by secondary changes in bone, and development of osteophytes, resulting in many cases in reduction in joint mobility and pain on movement.

Osteoarthritis of the lower limbs and spine may affect gait and balance. Arthritis of the hip leads to stiffness and restriction of hip movement and an antalgic gait. Arthritic knees cause pain and stiffness on movement, and may produce instability of the joint, leaving a joint that 'gives way', causing falls. Muscle weakness secondary to pain and stiffness in lower limb joints leads to further instability.

Spinal degenerative disease, which is also extremely common in the elderly, causes difficulties in two areas. In the cervical spine, spondylo-arthritis may produce interference with proprioception, gait disturbance because of cervical myelopathy, and occasionally may interfere with brain-stem vascular supply via the vertebral arteries. In the lumbar spine there may be restriction of spinal movements and pain and weakness in lower limbs because of nerve or root compression. All of these problems can lead to instability and falls.

Diseases which are associated with falls

These may relate to any system of the body, though there are particular types of problems that are more likely to be associated with falls than others. Any acute illness may present as a fall, and falling is one of the common non-specific presentations of acute ill-health in the elderly.

It is sometimes helpful to divide falls caused by specific diseases into those where consciousness is lost and those where it is not, though there is clearly some overlap between the two groups. In general, falls associated with loss of consciousness result from a small group of diseases, though it can sometimes be extremely difficult to determine the cause of loss of consciousness in an elderly subject. This topic is considered further in Chapter 6. The conditions discussed below are by no means an exhaustive list of diseases associated with falls, but include some of the commoner and more important problems which can cause falls.

Epilepsy

Epilepsy is a clinical diagnosis which depends largely on the history, and because the consciousness of the subject is interfered with during the event, he/she cannot provide a full account of what happened. If there is no witness, which is often the case for elderly people, the history will be incomplete. The differential diagnosis of loss of consciousness in the elderly is wide, and any event causing cerebral anoxia may be followed by a convulsion. Thus, the diagnosis of epilepsy in the elderly is a particularly problematic one. Even in a situation where syncopal episodes have been witnessed by trained staff, almost a third of events remain unexplained (Lipsitz et al., 1985).

Although studies of falls may attempt to exclude fits, an elderly person may forget the loss of consciousness and remember only the fall, or the carer may report that the person was 'found on the floor', and an assumption is made that a simple fall has occurred. It is thus difficult to know what proportion of falls are due to epilepsy. In a study of episodes of loss of consciousness in an elderly institutionalised population the one year incidence of syncope was 7 per cent, and of these only a very small proportion (4 per cent of those with syncope) were found to be due to 'seizure disorder', though 'obvious seizures in patients with known seizure disorders were excluded' (Lipsitz et al., 1985). Since the prevalence of falling in the very elderly, frail population studied (mean age 87 years) is likely to be of the order of 50 per cent per year, epilepsy would seem to account for a very small proportion of falls.

Studies of the incidence and prevalence of epilepsy carried out recently have demonstrated that epilepsy is commoner in those over 60 than in the population as a whole. Prevalence of epilepsy in the elderly is approximately 12 per 1000 (compared to 9 per 1000 for the population overall), and increases with increasing age. Incidence is again higher in older populations, with a sharper rise with age, ranging from 76/100 000 for those over 60 to 159/100 000 for those over 80, compared to a total population incidence of 69/100 000 (Tallis et al., 1991). Comparing these figures to figures for the prevalence of falling suggests that epilepsy probably accounts for only a few per cent of falls.

Parkinson's disease

People with Parkinson's disease fall with monotonous regularity. The typical gait changes experienced by those with Parkinsonism (stooped posture, festinant gait, shuffling) are a partial explanation of the propensity of such patients to fall. However, there does also seem to be a specific impairment of postural reflexes and righting reflexes as part of the disease, and some people develop these before the more typical features of Parkinson's disease such as rigidity, bradykinesia and tremor (Klawans and Topel, 1974). Postural hypotension, either because of an associated autonomic neuropathy or because of the hypotensive effect of antiparkinsonian medication (and commonly because of a combination of the two) may be another factor in the frequency of falls in those with Parkinson's disease.

Case report

A 72 year-old woman with a five year history of Parkinson's disease was referred for assessment of recurrent falls. She was taking small doses of an L-dopa/dopa-decarboxylase inhibitor combination, and an anticholinergic drug. She was also taking a thiazide diuretic for postural oedema and nitrazepam for night sedation. On examination she had marked bradykinesia and rigidity, and a postural drop in blood pressure of 40 mmHg associated with symptoms of light-headedness. Her anticholinergic medication was gradually reduced and stopped, her L-dopa combination treatment was increased and the diuretic was discontinued. She continued to have a milder degree of postural hypotension, but it was possible to control this (and her postural oedema) with compression stockings. Her mobility and independence improved, and the frequency of her falls was much reduced.

Cerebrovascular disease

Strokes have consistently been identified as a risk factor for falls in many studies. This is true both for those with persisting hemipareses and those whose neurological signs have resolved, so the tendency to fall is not purely due to overt neurological deficits. The more subtle disturbances of neurological functioning that strokes can cause appear to interfere with balance in ways that are not always fully understood. Where there is obvious limb weakness or sensory loss gait is often affected, and the reason for a predisposition to falls is clear. Sensory or visual inattention or neglect will produce a tendency to bump into or trip over things, and parietal lobe involvement may lead to problems with planning and carrying out complicated actions, increasing risk of falling during activity. Damage to frontal lobes may interfere with judgement resulting in risky actions being attempted. Brainstem and cerebellar strokes directly damage areas closely involved in maintenance of balance. All of these factors will contribute to an increased liability to falls in those with cerebrovascular disease.

Peripheral neuropathies

Sensory input via peripheral nerves is an important part of the proprioceptive information upon which maintenance of balance depends. People with sensory peripheral neuropathies therefore have a degree of interference with part of the balance feedback control system, though major problems with balance are unusual in the absence of other sensory problems, such as visual impairment. Motor peripheral neuropathies, causing lower limb weakness, can interfere with the efferent limb of the feedback loop and also tend to interfere with balance.

Myopathies

Any cause of lower limb weakness is associated with an increased risk of falling. The most common pattern of muscle weakness is a proximal myopathy, with weakness affecting the pelvic and shoulder girdles rather than the distal muscles. This causes difficulties getting up from a chair, and tends to produce a waddling gait. Because these common everyday movements are involved and altered, there is a risk of falling during day to day activities, and once a fall has occurred, the faller often has severe difficulty getting up from the floor.

Important causes of proximal myopathy in elderly subjects include osteomalacia, polymyalgia rheumatica, hypercalcaemia, hypo- and hyperthyroidism, polymyositis and dermatomyositis. Iatrogenic Cushings syndrome (which is much commoner than idiopathic Cushings disease or ectopic ACTH syndrome) is another well recognised cause of proximal muscle weakness. More generalised weakness may be the result of electrolyte imbalances such as hyponatraemia and hypokalaemia, both most commonly caused by treatment with diuretics.

Case report

An 80 year-old woman was admitted to hospital as an emergency having spent the night on the floor following a fall. She gave a history of several months of general aches and pains, depression, and difficulty getting up from a chair. Examination revealed moderate proximal muscle weakness, and pain on moving shoulders and hips. A clinical diagnosis of polymyalgia rheumatica was made and confirmed by an ESR of 98 mm in the first hour. Treatment with steroids produced a dramatic improvement in her symptoms within 48 hours. She had no further falls over 18 months follow-up.

Dementia

The cognitively impaired have been shown in a number of studies to be at greater risk of falling. Although this may partly be due to lack of insight into environmental dangers, and failure of compliance, either with medical treatment or with advice about safety, there also seems to be a specific problem with postural stability, perhaps because of organic damage to central balance mechanisms. Elderly people with dementia who develop behavioural problems are also quite likely to be given phenothiazines or other sedatives and tranquillisers, which contribute to their instability and risk of falling.

Cervical spondylosis

By the time they reach their 70s and 80s, most people have some degree of arthritis of the joints of the cervical spine. However, only a proportion of elderly people have symptoms referrable to these joint changes. There are four main syndromes associated with cervical spondylo-arthritis, of which three have important implications for risk of falling.

1. Disc degeneration and protrusion with bony overgrowth of the adjacent vertebrae can compress the cervical spine, particularly in those with a congenitally narrow spinal canal, leading to a progressive spastic paraparesis. This can interfere with gait and lead to falls.
2. Root compression because of lateral protrusion of discs or osteophytes produces pain and sensory symptoms in the affected root territory in the upper limb but does not increase risk of falling.
3. The joints of the cervical spine are rich in proprioceptive nerve endings, and provide much information about the position of the body in space and the relative positions of the head and body. Where movements of these joints are limited because of arthritis, the amount of proprioceptive information available to the balance system is reduced. This can result in a sensation of instability or 'dizziness', and particularly when there are other sensory problems, the ability to maintain balance and prevent falls may be impaired.
4. The vertebral arteries pass through foramina in the transverse processes of the cervical vertebrae, turning sharply backwards after leaving the atlas to enter the skull through the foramen magnum. They then join together to form the basilar artery. Branches from the vertebral and basilar arteries supply the brainstem. In a very small proportion of people with cervical spondylosis, osteophytes compress the vertebral arteries and interfere with the blood supply to the brainstem when extreme movements of the cervical spine are attempted. Vertigo may be produced, but almost invariably

other brainstem symptoms and signs also occur, such as double vision, slurring of speech, bilateral visual loss or unilateral weakness or sensory symptoms. A vague sensation of dizziness or instability on turning the head is rarely due to so-called 'vertebrobasilar insufficiency', and is more likely to be due to impaired sensory input from cervical spine proprioceptors.

Diabetes

The diabetic has numerous potential causes of falls. These include hypoglycaemia due to over-treatment with insulin or oral hypoglycaemics, peripheral or autonomic neuropathies, problems arising from associated ischaemic heart disease (such as cardiac arrhythmias or cardiac failure), peripheral vascular disease and strokes, and visual impairment because of diabetic retinopathy or cataracts. The problem with assessment of diabetics who have fallen is often not 'what caused the fall', but which of many potential causes was responsible.

Cardiac arrhythmias

There seem to be difficulties in assessing the role of cardiac arrhythmias in falls. Case reports of elderly people with falls who were found to have abnormalities on 24-hour ECG monitoring suggest that cardiac arrhythmias are common causes of falls (Gordon, 1978), but do not give enough information to estimate what proportion of falls is actually due to this problem. One study found that the number of accidents (mostly simple falls) in subjects known to have episodic cardiac arrhythmias was twice that in age- and sex-matched controls, though there was no significant increase in fracture rate (Nilsson and Abdon, 1980). In another study a third of patients with fractured neck of femur were found to have previously undiagnosed episodic cardiac arrhythmias on 24-hour ECG monitoring (Abdon and Nilsson, 1980). Serious episodic arrhythmias were found in 16.5 per cent of elderly people (who were age and sex matched controls for patients with suspected Stokes–Adams syndrome, rather than randomly selected controls), and were significantly commoner in those who had had attacks of dizziness or syncope (Abdon, 1981).

However, asymptomatic cardiac arrhythmias are common in the elderly (Rodrigues Dos Santos and Lye, 1980), and the relationship between arrhythmias and symptoms is not close even in those with symptoms of dizziness or syncope (Clarke et al., 1980). In a group of institutionalised elderly, the frequency of arrhythmias on 24-hour cardiac monitoring was the same in fallers as in matched non-fallers (Rosado et al., 1989). On balance, although cardiac arrhythmias can in some situations cause falls, the demonstration of an arrhythmia (other than one found whilst monitoring during the fall) does not necessarily prove that the cause of the fall was an arrhythmia.

Case report

A 76 year-old woman was referred to the outpatient clinic for assessment of blackouts. They had been occurring every few months for the last year. She attended clinic alone and history from her did not reveal any obvious precipitating factors, though she had mild stable angina, and she was otherwise well. A 24-hour ECG recording showed frequent ventricular ectopic beats and occasional pairs of ectopics, not associated with symptoms (she did not have a blackout during taping). In the absence of any obvious alternative explanation for her blackouts, she was started on antiarrhythmic medication. On review she reported that her blackouts had continued unabated. An alternative antiarrhythmic was tried, with no effect. At the fourth or fifth review her husband attended clinic with her, and when questioned about her blackouts he reported that they were preceded by stereotyped lipsmacking movements, and followed by drowsiness and confusion for a few hours. Treatment with anti-epileptic medication stopped her blackouts completely.

Carotid sinus syndrome

Carotid sinus syndrome can produce symptoms of syncope, falls and dizziness due to episodic impairment of cerebral perfusion. There is an exaggerated response to stimulation of baroreceptor reflex pathways when pressure is applied to the carotid sinus, resulting in transient reflex asystole and vasodepression. Increasing sensitivity to carotid sinus massage seems to occur with age, and may cause a proportion of falls and dizziness reported by the elderly. In a group of patients referred for investigation of falls, dizziness and syncope, 23 per cent had carotid sinus syndrome with no other identifiable cause for their symptoms (Kenny and Traynor, 1991).

Environment and falls

Environmental factors are important in maintaining the independence of elderly people. They are also important as causes of falls, though separating intrinsic and extrinsic causes of falls is difficult. In general, it seems that environmental factors are a sole or major cause of between a third and a half of falls resulting in injury (Morfitt, 1983; Citron, 1985), though such falls are a small proportion of falls overall. The proportion in which environmental factors predominate is probably less in the very elderly for whom intrinsic factors are commoner causes of falls. Environmental factors include such common events as tripping over uneven paving stones or slipping on ice, but factors reported in one study of falls indicate that the elderly sometimes have exciting lives, being chased by bulls, falling off dressing tables and being knocked over by gas boiler explosions (Clark, 1968).

The environment and intrinsic factors interact to increase risk of falling. For example when vision is poor, low lighting levels exacerbate the effects of visual loss (Cullinan et al., 1979), and this may be particularly important for negotiating stairs because of the patterns of light produced (Archea, 1985). Those with gait problems may find that these are made worse by carpeted floors.

Studies of falls in hospitals or residential care institutions mention the importance of staffing levels (Blake and Morfitt, 1986) but very low staffing levels may be associated with fewer falls because patient activity is discouraged (Morris and Isaacs, 1980). Falls in hospital are sometimes associated with ward furniture, such as commodes, cotsides and 'geriatric chairs'. These issues are discussed further in Chapter 8.

There is some evidence that environmental temperature affects the risk of falling, at least in women (Campbell et al., 1988), though this may occur only in thin or undernourished women (Bastow et al., 1983) perhaps because of a relationship between nutritional state and thermoregulation. There is no doubt that frank hypothermia increases likelihood of falls because of effects on conscious level and control of movement. A fall may also be the cause of hypothermia if the faller is injured or unable to get up independently. Apart from the possible relationship between nutritional state, thermoregulation and falls, poor nutrition has not been shown to be associated with an increased incidence of falls. Community-living elderly with a history of recent falls had no objective evidence of poor nutritional state compared to non-fallers (Downton and Andrews, 1991)

The environment, both inside and outside the home, is a minefield of potential dangers for those with a tendency to fall. The opportunities presented for tripping, slipping, stumbling and overbalancing during the activities of daily life are endless, and people are often perverse in their determination to continue to put themselves at risk of falling by carrying out such activities. This at least is the view of many formal and informal carers of elderly people – the elderly themselves often reckon that the risk of falling is a price worth paying to maintain their independence and self-esteem.

The reasons that old people fall, and the factors that influence their risk of falling, are extremely numerous. In the vast majority of cases, there is not one single 'cause' of a fall, but a combination of factors, including age-related physiological changes, one or more pathological factors, and interactions between intrinsic and environmental factors. It follows, therefore, that determining the cause or causes of an individual fall, or investigation of the tendency of an elderly person to fall is correspondingly complicated and difficult. It is, however, always worth attempting to find the cause of the fall, because there is almost always some scope to reduce the risk of further falls, even in the very frailest elderly. The diagnostic and therapeutic nihilism which falls often induce is unjustified and unjustifiable.

References

Abdon, N.J. (1981). Frequency and distribution of long-term ECG-recorded cardiac arrhythmias in an elderly population. *Acta Med Scand.* **209:** 175–183.

Abdon, N.J. and Nilsson, B.E. (1980). Episodic cardiac arrhythmia and femoral neck fracture. *Acta Med Scand.* **208:** 73–76.

Archea, J.C. (1985). Environmental factors associated with stair accidents by the elderly. *Clin Geriatr Med.* **1:** 555–568.

Bastow, M.D., Rawlings, J. and Allison, S.P. (1983). Undernutrition, hypothermia, and injury in elderly women with fractured femur: an injury response to altered metabolism? *Lancet.* **1:** 143–146.

Blake, C. and Morfitt, J.M. (1986). Falls and staffing in a residential home for elderly people. *Public Health.* **100:** 385–391.

Blessed, G., Tomlinson, B.E. and Roth, M. (1968). The association between quantitative measures of dementia and of senile change in the cerebral grey matter of elderly subjects. *Br J Psychiatry.* **114:** 787–811.

Brocklehurst, J.C., Robertson, D. and James-Groom, P. (1982). Clinical correlates of sway in old age – sensory modalities. *Age Ageing.* **11:** 1–10.

Broe, G.A., Akhtar, A.J., Andrews, G.R., Caird, F.I., Gilmore, A.J.J. and McLennan, W.J. (1976). Neurological disorders in the elderly at home. *J Neurol Neurosurg Psychiatry.* **39:** 362–366.

Caird, F.I., Andrews, G.R. and Kennedy, R.D. (1973). Effect of posture on blood pressure in the elderly. *Br Heart J.* **35:** 527–530.

Campbell, A.J., Spears, G.F.S., Borrie, M.J. and Fitzgerald, J.L. (1988). Falls, elderly women and the cold. *Gerontology.* **34:** 205–208.

Citron, N. (1985). Femoral neck fractures: are some preventable? *Ergonomics.* **28:** 993–997.

Clark, A.N.G. (1968). Factors in fracture of the female femur. A clinical study of the environmental, physical, medical and preventative aspects of this injury. *Geront Clin.* **10:** 257–270.

Clarke, P.I., Glasser, S.P. and Spoto, E. (1980). Arrhythmias detected by ambulatory monitoring. Lack of correlation with symptoms of dizziness and syncope. *Chest.* **77:** 722–725.

Collins, K.J., Exton-Smith, A.N., James, M.H. and Oliver, D.J. (1980). Functional changes in autonomic nervous responses with ageing. *Age Ageing.* **9:** 17–24.

Cullinan, T.R., Silver, J.H., Gould, E.S. and Irvine, D. (1979). Visual disability and home lighting. *Lancet.* **1:** 642–644.

DeVries, H.A., Wiswell, R.A., Romero, G.T. and Heckathonne, E. (1985). Changes with age in monosynaptic reflexes elicited by mechanical and electrical stimulation. *Am J Phys Med.* **64:** 71–81.

Dorfman, L.J. and Bosley, T.M. (1979). Age-related changes in peripheral and central nerve conduction in man. *Neurology.* **29:** 38–44.

Downton, J.H. and Andrews, K. (1991). Prevalence, characteristics and factors associated with falls among the elderly living at home. *Aging.* **3:** 219–228.

Fiatarone, M.A., Marks, E.C., Ryan, N.D., Meredith, C.N., Lipsitz, L.A. and Evans, W.J. (1990). High intensity strength training in nonegenarians. Effects on skeletal muscle. *JAMA.* **263:** 3029–3034.

Gerson, L.W., Jarjoura, D. and McCord, G. (1989). Risk of imbalance in elderly people with impaired hearing or vision. *Age Ageing.* **18:** 31–34.

Gordon, M. (1978). Occult cardiac arrhythmias associated with falls and dizziness in the elderly: detection by Holter monitoring. *J Am Geriatr Soc.* **26:** 418–423.

Gribbin, B., Pickering, T.G., Sleight, P. and Peto, R. (1971). Effect of age and high blood pressure on baroreflex sensitivity in man. *Circ Res.* **29:** 424–431.

Hogan, D.B., Berman, P., Fox, R.A., Hubley-Kozey, C.L., Turnbull, G. and Wall, J. (1987). Idiopathic gait disorders in the elderly. *Clin Rehab*. **1:** 17–22.

Impallomeni, M., Kenny, R.A., Flynn, M.D., Kraenzlin, M. and Pallis, C.A. (1984). The elderly and their ankle jerks. *Lancet*. **1:** 670–672.

Kenny, R.A. and Traynor, G. (1991). Carotid sinus syndrome – clinical characteristics in elderly patients. *Age Ageing*. **20:** 449–454.

Kirshen, A.J., Cape, R.D.T., Hayes, H.C. and Spencer, J.D. (1984). Postural sway and cardiovascular parameters associated with falls in the elderly. *J Clin Exp Gerontol*. **6:** 291–307.

Klawans, H.L. and Topel, J.L. (1974). Parkinsonism as a falling sickness. *JAMA*. **230:** 1555–1557.

Lipsitz, L.A., Nyquist, R.P., Wei, J.Y. and Rowe, J.W. (1983). Postprandial reduction in blood pressure in the elderly. *N Engl J Med*. **309:** 81–83.

Lipsitz, L.A., Wei, J.Y. and Rowe, J.W. (1985). Syncope in an elderly institutionalised population: prevalence, incidence and associated risk. *Q J Med*. **55:** 45–54.

MacLennan, W.J., Timothy, J.I. and Hall, M.R.P. (1980). Vibration sense, proprioception and ankle reflexes in old age. *J Clin Exp Gerontol*. **2:** 159–171.

Maki, B.E., Holliday, P.J., Fernie, G.R. (1990). Aging and postural control. A comparison of spontaneous- and induced-sway balance tests. *J Am Geriatr Soc*. **38:** 1–9.

Milne, J.S. (1979). Longitudinal studies of vision in older people. *Age Ageing*. **8:** 160–166.

Morfitt, J.M. (1983). Falls in old people at home: intrinsic versus environmental factors in causation. *Public Health*. **97:** 115–120.

Morris, E.V. and Isaacs, B. (1980). The prevention of falls in a geriatric hospital. *Age Ageing*. **9:** 181–185.

Nebes, R.D. (1978). Vocal verses manual response as a determinant of age difference in simple reaction time. *J Gerontol*. **33:** 884–889.

Nelson, P., Hughes, S., Virjee, S., Beresford, H., Murray, C., Watson, E. and Sandercock, P. (1991). Walking speed as a measure of disability. *Care of the Elderly*. **3 (3):** 125–126.

Nilsson, B.E., Abdon, N.J. (1980). Episodic cardiac arrhythmia and accident rate. *Acta Med Scand*. **208:** 69–71.

Norre, M.E., Forrez, G. and Beckers, A. (1987). Posturography measuring instability in vestibular dysfunction in the elderly. *Age Ageing*. **16:** 89–93.

Oosterveld, W.J. (1983). Changes in vestibular function with increasing age. In *Hearing and Balance in the Elderly,* Hinchcliffe, R., (ed.). Edinburgh: Churchill Livingstone.

Prakash, C. and Stern, G. (1973). Neurological signs in the elderly. *Age Ageing*. **2:** 24–27.

Rickli, R. and Busch, S. (1986). Motor performance of women as a function of age and physical activity level. *J Gerontol*. **41:** 645–649.

Robinson, B.J., Johnson, R.H., Lambie, D.G. and Palmer, K.T. (1983). Do elderly patients with an excessive fall in blood pressure on standing have evidence of autonomic failure? *Clin Sci*. **64:** 587–591.

Rodrigues Dos Santos, A.G., Lye, M. (1980). Transient cardiac arrhythmias in healthy elderly individuals: how relevant are they? *J Clin Exp Gerontol*. **2:** 245–258.

Rosado, J.A., Rubenstein, L.Z., Robbins, A.S., Heng, M.K., Schulman, B.L. and Josephson, K.R. (1989). The value of Holter monitoring in evaluating the elderly patient who falls. *J Am Geriatr Soc*. **37:** 430–434.

Smith, S.A. and Fasler, J.J. (1983). Age-related changes in autonomic function – relationship with postural hypotension. *Age Ageing*. **12:** 206–210.

Spirduso, W.W. (1975). Reaction and movement time as as function of age and physical activity level. *J Gerontol.* **30:** 435–440.

Sudarsky, L. and Ronthal, M. (1983). Gait disorders among elderly patients. A survey study of 50 patients. *Arch Neurol.* **40:** 740–743.

Tallis, R., Hall, G., Craig, I. and Dean, A. (1991). How common are epileptic seizures in old age? *Age Ageing.* **20:** 442–448.

Teno, J., Kiel, D.P. and Mor, V. (1990). Multiple stumbles: a risk factor for falls in community-dwelling elderly. A prospective study. *J Am Geriatrics Soc.* **38:** 1321–1325.

Whipple, R.H., Wolfson, L.I. and Amerman, P.M. (1987). The relationship of knee and ankle weakness to falls in Nursing Home residents: an isokinetic study. *J Am Geriatr Soc.* **35:** 13–20.

Wolfson, L.I., Whipple, R., Amerman, P. and Kleinberg, A. (1986). Stressing the postural response. A quantitative method for testing balance. *J Am Geriatr Soc.* **34:** 845–850.

Wolfson, L.I., Whipple, R., Amerman, P. and Tobin, J.N. (1990). Gait assessment in the elderly: a gait abnormality rating scale and its relation to falls. *J Gerontol.* **45:** M12–M19.

Wollner, L., McCarthy, S.T., Soper, N.D.W. and Macy, D.J. (1979). Failure of cerebral autoregulation as a cause of brain dysfunction in the elderly. *Br Med J.* **1:** 1117–1118.

Chapter 6

Dizziness and syncope

Elderly people who fall quite commonly comment, either spontaneously, or when asked to account for their fall, that they felt 'dizzy'. This is often interpreted by someone with medical training as implying vertigo, setting in train treatment with so-called 'vestibular sedatives' in an attempt to suppress the 'dizziness' and prevent further falls. This is one of many instances where lay and medical understanding of terms differs.

Dizziness is very much a 'Humpty-Dumpty' word, which when used by the elderly to describe their experiences means what they want it to mean, and not necessarily what the doctor understands it to mean. 'Dizziness', like 'indigestion', means different things to different people. When someone complains of feeling dizzy, this may imply any one (or more) of a wide range of subjective sensations, mirrored by the range of synonyms for such symptoms (Table 6.1). This is by no means an exhaustive list, and terms vary geographically. A Finnish study of dizziness also found symptoms such as 'spots before the eyes', staggering, loss of balance, a feeling of falling, heaviness or confusion in the head and buzzing in the ears being included by patients in descriptions of dizziness (Orma and Koskenoja, 1957a). Patients with dizziness commonly experience more than one type of symptom.

Table 6.1 Synonyms for dizzy and dizziness.

Lightheaded
Mazy
Giddy
Drunk/intoxicated
'Swimmy'
Floating
Dazed
Queer (as in 'I came over all queer')
Ataxia
Vertigo
Dysequilibrium
Faintness
Imbalance
Grey-out
Confusion

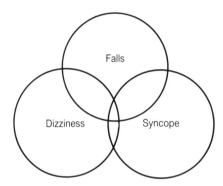

Fig. 6.1 Overlap between falls, dizziness and syncope

Some of the symptoms of dizziness imply loss, or near loss of consciousness, and correspond to the medical term syncope. However, people are sometimes unsure whether they blacked-out completely, or even whether they blacked-out at all. Although we can often convince ourselves that in an individual case we are or are not dealing with syncope, in reality there is an overlap between dizziness and syncope (Fig. 6.1) and the same underlying causes may produce either symptom. That is the reason for dealing with both dizziness and syncope in one chapter, as a separation between the two symptoms is to some extent artificial and arbitrary. Because of the confusion of terminology, I shall use dizziness as a non-specific description of all of these symptoms, and the more specific synonyms (such as vertigo, syncope, dysequilibrium, etc.) where specific diseases or pathophysiological events are being discussed.

The subjective nature of the symptom of dizziness means that it is impossible to know whether the experience that someone is describing corresponds to the experience that the listener has experienced and/or understands by the term. Unlike a symptom such as 'angina' which is described in a fairly consistent way by most sufferers, dizziness appears to be experienced in many different ways, some of which seem to be virtually and genuinely indescribable. In an attempt to understand what the sufferer is experiencing, we may offer him/her alternative descriptions which fit with our understanding of the potential disease processes, but paradoxically that may increase the canyon of misunderstanding between us.

True vertigo (by which is meant an illusion or hallucination of movement, either of the patient or of his/her surroundings) is usually rather clearer than the other types of dizziness, and since almost everyone has experienced a mild version of the sensation in childhood when getting off a rotating roundabout, or stopping after spinning round, it is usually possible to determine whether the symptom is vertigo. Severe acute vertigo, such as that due to acute vestibular failure is an extremely distressing symptom. '[A] labyrinthine disturbance may make [patients] feel that the end of the world has arrived and ... in the acutest phase of their distress, they wish that it had' (Cawthorne, 1945). The symptom of vertigo seems to more consistently described by sufferers than other types of dizziness, but the other types of symptoms are considerably more difficult to define and understand.

What is 'dizziness?'

The sensation of vertigo arises because of mismatch of sensory information arriving at the brainstem. Information from the vestibular labyrinth tells the brainstem that movement is occurring, whilst information from the eyes and somatosensors tells the brainstem that movement is not occurring. The more indefinite types of dizziness may also arise from sensory mismatch, for instance in the symptoms experienced by those with multiple sensory impairments. Symptoms of dizziness fall into four main groups (Drachmann and Hart, 1972).

1. An hallucination of movement of self or environment, i.e. true vertigo.
2. Symptoms associated with some degree of impairment of consciousness, and presumably related to transient global (or occasionally focal) impairment of cerebral circulation, i.e. near syncope or syncope.
3. Sensations of dysequilibrium.
4. 'Other', covering in general the more non-specific and difficult to describe subjective sensations.

In the first, and to some extent the second, categories, there is a fairly close relationship between symptoms and pathophysiology. In general, however, the symptom of dizziness is often very vague and can result from diseases in any system of the body, from psychological problems, or indeed from physiological sensations.

How common is dizziness?

Partly because the symptom covers such a wide range of sensations, it is a frequent complaint amongst the elderly. Subjective symptoms of dizziness are reported to affect between a third and a half of the elderly population but it is not always clear what sorts of dizziness are being experienced by the subjects of those studies. Various different terms are used in different studies, not all of which are very clear or unambiguous.

One of the earliest community studies of the elderly and their health and functional state reported that 52 per cent of the subject group (aged 65+) had had 'vertigo', though it is unlikely that this meant true rotatory vertigo. There was an increasing prevalence of the symptom with age (Sheldon, 1948). Amongst a randomly selected population of people of pensionable age in Sheffield in the 1950s, 56 per cent (48 per cent of men and 62 per cent of women) complained of 'vertigo' (by which was meant either a sensation of rotation or a more non-specific symptom). These symptoms were more often occasional than frequent, but became increasingly common with increasing age (Droller, 1955). In the Newcastle community study (Evans, 1990), 13 per cent of those aged 75 and over had experienced rotatory dizziness, and 30 per cent had had non-rotatory dizziness (some had had both). A community study of subjects aged 75 and over found that almost half suffered occasional or frequent subjective feelings of postural imbalance or dizziness (Downton and Andrews, 1990).

Amongst a representative sample of 75 year olds in Goteborg, Sweden, 40 per cent of women and 30 per cent of men complained of various symptoms of 'postural disturbances', of which the commonest was unsteadiness, affecting almost three quarters of those with complaints. A sensation of personal rotation accounted for about a quarter of symptoms and vertigo for a smaller percentage. Many subjects had more than one symptom (Sixt and Landahl, 1987). In a large community based American study, 34 per cent of subjects (aged 60+) complained of some degree of dizziness, and in 19 per cent it was of sufficient severity to result in a visit to a physician, to require medication, or to interfere with the subject's life 'a lot' (Sloane et al., 1989). Another American community screening programme found that 14 per cent of women and 11 per cent of men aged 65+ reported dizziness, with prevalence increasing with increasing age (Hale et al., 1986).

Amongst those who present to medical attention following their fall, a larger percentage appear to have suffered dizziness or faintness (Lucht, 1971). This may reflect a greater likelihood of injury if consciousness is impaired or lost (Kapoor et al., 1986a). In the United States, dizziness is a presenting complaint in about 4 per cent of consultations with primary care practices in those aged over 65 years (Sloane, 1989). The proportion increases with age and dizziness is substantially commoner in women than men, particularly in the very elderly.

The relationship between dizziness and falls

A variable proportion of fallers describe their falls as being due to dizziness. Interpreting the data available is difficult because of the different symptoms which are covered by the term. In Sheldon's 1948 study, a quarter of those who had had falls ascribed their falls to 'vertigo', but a more recent community study of those of 75 and over found that only 7 per cent of falls were due to dizziness, and there was only a weak relationship between symptoms of dizziness and a history of falls (Downton and Andrews, 1990) The Newcastle study found no association between rotatory dizziness and falling, but non-rotatory dizziness was associated with falling, occurring in 30 per cent of fallers compared with 22 per cent of non-fallers (Prudham and Evans, 1981).

Causes of dizziness

Most studies considering the causes of dizziness in the elderly have been based on patients referred either to specialist 'dizziness clinics' or to ear, nose and throat (ENT) clinics, rather than unselected elderly. Dizziness is a common reason for referral to an ENT clinic, accounting for about a third of referrals (Belal and Glorig, 1986). However, there seems to be quite a marked variation in the frequency with which various diagnoses are found in different studies, partly reflecting different diagnostic pathways, some of which seem to be fairly subjective. The proportion in which a 'specific' or 'definitive' diagnosis can be made varies from 21 per cent (Belal and Glorig, 1986) to 84 per cent (Baloh et al., 1989). Peripheral vestibular problems seem in most cases to be the commonest cause of vertigo, accounting for between a quarter and a half of patients (Drachmann and Hart, 1972; Overstall et al., 1981; Baloh et al., 1989), but one cannot help gaining the impression that observers find the conditions that they are looking for. In most studies there is a group that remains 'undiagnosed', sometimes because no abnormalities can be demonstrated on examination and specialised testing, sometimes because there are 'too many' abnormalities found to allow allocation to a specific diagnostic category. It is not uncommon for dizzy patients to have more than one disease or diagnosis accounting for their symptoms (Baloh et al., 1989), as well as having more than one type of dizziness.

There are differences of opinion about how useful history alone is in indicating the cause of dizziness. Some feel that a diagnosis can be reached primarily on the history in a majority of dizzy subjects, particularly in those in whom a definitive diagnosis can be made (Sloane and Baloh, 1989), whereas others feel that history alone (using a standardised questionnaire) correlates poorly with vestibular testing (Spitzer, 1990).

Interpreting studies of dizziness is complicated by the lack of standardisation of diagnostic categories and even lack of definition of terms. In a study with a somewhat subjective separation of patients with dysequilibrium of ageing (presbyastasis) into various different groups depending on whether their dizziness was constant, positional, orthostatic or 'unclassified', there did not appear to be a clear distinction between the groups on various audiological and other investigations (Belal and Glorig, 1986).

It has been suggested that the majority (>90 per cent) of dizziness in the elderly is postural dizziness, by which is meant non-vertiginous dizziness occurring in connection with movement of body or head, or with specific positions (Orma and Koskenoja, 1957b). However, this has not been supported by studies of subjects attending ENT clinics. Of those who were classified as suffering from 'dysequilibrium of ageing' 19 per cent had positional symptoms and 5 per cent had orthostatic symptoms, but in 57 per cent, symptoms were constant (Belal and Glorig, 1986). Another study reported a 60:40 split between episodic and continuous dizziness. Forty-two per cent of the subjects experienced vertigo, 28 per cent dysequilibrium, 13 per cent presyncopal lightheadedness, and 17 per cent 'other' symptoms (Sloane and Baloh, 1989).

The main causes of dizziness (in those referred to specialist ENT or dizziness clinics at least) appear to be peripheral vestibular disorders (frequently benign paroxysmal positional vertigo), central vestibular dysfunction and other central neurological disorders, and multiple sensory impairments, though a variable proportion of dizzy patients have psychological problems underlying their complaints (Downton and Andrews, 1990).

The main conclusion to be drawn from studies looking at types of dizziness is that there is no consensus of opinion, perhaps reflecting the difficulties of defining and classifying such vague and subjective sensations. However, causes of dizziness can be divided into several groups that to some extent mirror the main types of symptoms experienced (Table 6.2). However, as already mentioned, an individual patient may have more than one type of symptom and more than one cause for their symptom(s).

Although in real life, patients and their symptoms often cannot be neatly categorised, consideration of the causes of dizziness is helped by separating the symptom into the four main groups discussed above. In each group there are conditions which are common and/or well defined which cause the particular type of dizziness.

Table 6.2 Causes of dizziness.

1. True vertigo
    a) Peripheral vestibular problems
        BPPV
        Menières disease
        'Vestibular neuronitis'
        Toxic damage, e.g. aminoglycosides
        Chronic suppurative otitis media
    b) Central vestibular problems
        Acoustic neuroma
        Brainstem disorders, e.g. CVA, VBI, MS
    c) Central nervous system disorders
        Cerebellar disorders
        Epilepsy
        Migraine
2. Syncope or near-syncope – see later part of chapter
3. Dysequilibrium
    a) Somatosensory problems
        Peripheral neuropathies
        Cervical spondylosis
    b) Visual disorders
    c) Multiple sensory deficits
    d) Drug intoxication, e.g. alcohol, phenytoin, phenothiazines, benzodiazepines
    e) Psychological, e.g. hyperventilation, anxiety, depression
4. Other
    More difficult to tie down, but particularly likely to be partly or wholly due to multiple sensory deficits and/or psychological factors

Vertigo

If a patient complains of true vertigo, a sensation of rotation of self or environment, this limits the site of the problem to three main areas: peripheral vestibular (the vestibular labyrinth and vestibular nerve), central vestibular (the vestibular nuclei within the brain stem), and occasionally other areas of the central nervous system.

Peripheral vestibular problems

1. Benign paroxysmal positional vertigo (BPPV)

This is a syndrome with clear-cut symptoms, signs and findings on otological examination (Baloh et al., 1987). It produces episodes of vertigo, typically induced by such manoeuvres as turning over in bed, bending over and straightening up, or extending the neck to look up or reach for an object on a high shelf. Individual episodes never last more than a minute, but a flurry of episodes may leave a longer lasting, less specific feeling of dizziness. Bouts of vertigo are intermixed with various periods of remission.

The mean age of onset is in the mid-50s, but no age group is exempt. About half the time the condition appears to follow identifiable vestibular problems, such as trauma or 'vestibular neuronitis', the remainder being idiopathic. It is slightly more common in women than men, particularly in the idiopathic group.

Diagnosis can be confirmed by performing provocative tests (the Hallpike manoeuvre – Fig. 6.2) which produce torsional nystagmus (and usually vertigo in addition) after a latent interval of a few seconds. The nystagmus lasts less than a minute and fatigues (i.e. becomes more difficult to demonstrate and lasts a shorter time) on repeat testing. If there is no latent interval before onset of nystagmus and no fatiguing with repeat testing, then BPPV is not the cause, and a central vestibular lesion is likely to be present. BPPV is thought to be due to the presence of calcium carbonate crystals within the posterior semicircular canal. Movement of particles within the endolymph stimulates the vestibular neurones resulting in vertigo and nystagmus.

2. Menière's disease

This is a disease characterised by tinnitus, hearing loss and episodic vertigo which begins in middle life. With the passage of time, attacks of vertigo become less pronounced, but hearing loss and tinnitus are more prominent. Once the episodic vertigo has subsided, patients may be left with a more continuous feeling of imbalance and dizziness. Menières disease is probably over-diagnosed in the elderly.

3. 'Vestibular neuronitis'

This is a clinical syndrome rather than a diagnosis and is characterised by sudden onset of vertigo, often associated with nausea and vomiting, which

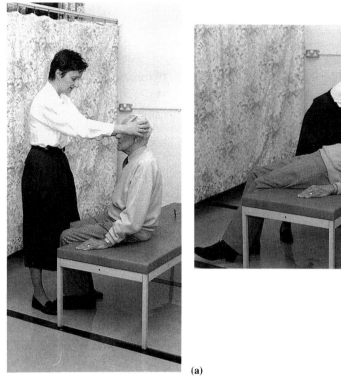

(b)

(a)

Fig. 6.2   The Hallpike manoeuvre to elicit positional nystagmus. Warn the subject that he is to be positioned with his head hanging down over the edge of the couch before carrying out the manoeuvre.

(a)   the subject sits looking at the tester to fix his gaze
(b)   the subject's head is turned gently and he is rapidly laid down whilst the tester watches for the development of nystagmus (see text). The subject's head should be hanging approximately 45° below the horizontal and rotated 45° to one side

lasts for several weeks, gradually diminishing before it settles completely. The aetiology is unclear, and may in some cases be due to viral infection, though in the elderly the majority are probably vascular. Investigation shows no hearing loss but evidence of unilaterally impaired vestibular function. Elderly victims of vestibular neuronitis are commonly left with mild episodic (or occasionally continuous) dizziness, and the syndrome may be the precursor of BPPV.

4. Toxic damage

There are a number of drugs which are specifically ototoxic, such as aminoglycosides, loop diuretics, quinine and salicylates, which may cause vertigo, though deafness is a more common sequel.

5. Chronic middle ear problems

For reasons that are not always clear, patients with chronic middle ear problems sometimes suffer from episodic vertigo. Sometimes the mechanism is apparent, such as in those with chronic suppurative otitis media, when direct invasion into the inner ear can occur, but even impacted wax in the external ear may cause intermittent vertigo.

Central vestibular and other central nervous system problems

Brainstem disorders such as brainstem strokes or multiple sclerosis may affect the vestibular nuclei and their connections in the brainstem, causing vertigo. Transient impairment of vertebrobasilar circulation has frequently been blamed for episodic dizziness (so-called 'vertebrobasilar insufficiency'), but is unlikely to be the cause in the absence of other evidence of brainstem dysfunction such as diplopia, dysarthria, bilateral visual loss, etc., particularly when the dizziness is of the non-specific type.

Central nervous system disorders (other than brainstem problems) that produce true vertigo are limited, and the mechanism is often unclear. Vertigo may sometimes be part of the aura of epilepsy, and cerebellar disorders can produce vertigo rather than just instability.

Case report

A 78 year-old man was admitted to hospital as an emergency because of dizziness, vomiting and inability to stand. These symptoms had appeared five days previously and had remained stable since them. An examination he had nystagmus to both sides and on upward gaze, dysarthria and bilateral limb ataxia. Three days after admission he developed a right hemiplegia. A computed tomographic (CT) brain scan was carried out, which demonstrated an infarct in the region of the left caudate.

Syncope and near syncope are discussed in the second part of this chapter.

Dysequilibrium

Common causes of dysequilibrium in the elderly fall into three main groups; sensory impairments, drug intoxication and psychological problems.

1. Sensory impairments

Interference with the sensory inputs on which balance depends can result in symptoms of imbalance, though because of redundancy of information, single losses are usually symptomatic only when balance is exceptionally stressed. In the elderly there is commonly a degree of impairment in several sensory inputs and it is this combination that results in the frequent complaints of dysequilibrium in this age group. Peripheral neuropathies, somatosensory impairment (for instance due to arthritis in the cervical spine or other joints), and visual disorders, either singly or in combination can result in symptoms of imbalance. Elderly people with multiple sensory deficits are particularly likely to have balance symptoms.

2. Drug intoxication

Many drugs can produce symptoms of dysequilibrium. The most obvious ones are those which are centrally acting, such as benzodiazepines, antidepressants and phenothiazines. It is worth remembering that Stemetil (prochlorperazine), commonly prescribed for 'dizziness' is a phenothiazine and can itself produce imbalance. Several other groups of drugs which are commonly prescribed for the elderly can be associated with instability and dizziness, including diuretics and non-steroidal anti-inflammatory drugs (Goodwin and Regan, 1982; Hale et al., 1984)

3. Psychological problems

Complaints of dysequilibrium (and dizziness generally) are a common symptom of anxiety in old people. In some cases the symptoms are mediated through hyperventilation. It is well recognised that depression may present with somatic symptoms and although these symptoms may be definite and localised, such as pain in various sites, they may also be more vague and diffuse. Continuous vague dysequilibrium or dizziness is commonly due to depression.

Less specific symptoms of 'dizziness'

It is often more difficult to pin down the cause of such ill-defined and vague symptoms. In many cases the cause seems to be a combination of abnormalities which are in themselves minor, particularly affecting the sensory system or cardiovascular system. Once again, psychological ill health is a common underlying factor. Drug treatment with psychoactive medication may cause non-specific feelings of dissociation which may be described as dizziness, and benzodiazepines seem to be particularly prone to do this. Unfortunately benzodiazepine withdrawal syndromes may also include similar symptoms.

Case report

A 70 year-old woman was referred to the outpatient clinic for assessment of dizziness. When she arrived at clinic she informed the consultant geriatrician that her symptoms had now settled. As a result of publicity in the newspapers about the side effects of triazolam, she had stopped the triazolam night sedation that she had been taking for several years, and within a day or two her symptoms of 'dizziness' (which on further questioning she described as a sensation of feeling distant and unstable) had disappeared.

Assessment of the dizzy patient

History

This is the first, and often the most important step in assessing the dizzy patient. The difficulties involved in conveying and understanding the often vague and imprecise symptoms subsumed by the term 'dizziness' have been mentioned above, but it is crucial to try to understand which type of sensation is being described. Although the ideal would be a description untainted by leading questions (which cannot avoid affecting the description) it is usually necessary to prompt the sufferer.

An important point to ascertain is the character of the sensation. Was it a sensation of rotation of self or environment, implying vertigo? Was it a sensation of lightheadedness, a feeling of being about to faint? Was it a sensation of dysequilibrium (which often seems to be associated with a feeling of being 'pulled' or 'pushed' to one side, or sometimes backwards or forwards)? Was it a less definite, less describable sensation than any of these?

The next important aspect is duration of symptoms, particularly individual attacks, and duration of attacks is particularly useful if vertigo has occurred. Vertigo lasting for a few seconds is probably physiological; the vertigo of BPPV lasts for a few minutes. Menières disease causes episodes of vertigo lasting for a few hours, whereas an attack lasting for days to weeks (usually

Table 6.3 Assessment of dizziness.

History
    Character – rotational/dysequilibrium/light-headedness/other
    Duration – seconds/minutes/hours/days/persistent
    Positional symptoms?
    Postural symptoms?
    Associated symptoms – otological/neurological
    General health
    Past medical history
    Drug history
    Social history
    Psychological symptoms

Examination
    Cranial nerves
    Cerebellar function
    Neck movements
    Positional tests (for BPPV)
    Ears
    BP lying and standing

gradually diminishing) suggests acute labyrinthine dysfunction such as 'vestibular neuronitis'.

The effect of position or posture on symptoms should be asked about, particularly whether specific movements or positions precipitate dizziness (standing from sitting or lying, turning the head, bending, looking up, turning over in bed, etc.). The presence of other symptoms suggesting ear disease is important, particularly if the symptom is vertigo. The cardinal symptoms of ear disease are hearing loss, tinnitus, local pain and discharge from the ear, and their presence in combination with vertigo suggests a peripheral vestibular problem. Other neurological symptoms should be sought and if present raise the possibility of central nervous system disease causing the dizziness.

Inquiries about past medical history and general health should be made, and medication taken regularly or intermittently should be ascertained. Finally, some attempt should be made to assess psychological health, and the effect of the patients symptoms on his/her everyday life.

Examination

In some cases specialised otological tests may be required, but many patients can be assessed on the basis of a full history and a simple, but careful, examination. Every elderly patient complaining of dizziness of whichever type should have a full medical examination, but there are particular aspects which should be covered carefully. Neurological examination is important, particularly looking for evidence of brainstem dysfunction, cerebellar problems or evidence of peripheral neuropathy.

Nystagmus is an important physical sign to identify. The presence of horizontal sawtooth nystagmus implies a peripheral vestibular or cerebellar problem, whereas any other type implies a central neurological lesion. There are a couple of simple tests which demonstrate the integrity of the brainstem and cerebellar control of conjugate eye movements. The pendulum test involves merely swinging a pendulum in front of the patients eyes and watching eye movements. There should be smooth pursuit of the pendulum by both eyes. Optokinetic nystagmus can be simply demonstrated using a tape measure by unrolling it in front of the patients eyes, and the nystagmus which is provoked should be the same in both directions. Cerebellar function is tested using the finger-nose test, rapid alternating movements and by observing the gait for truncal ataxia.

If the history suggests BPPV, specific positional tests (the Hallpike manoeuvre) may demonstrate diagnostic symptoms and signs. The characteristic signs are a latent period before onset of nystagmus and vertigo, and fatiguing of the signs on repeat testing.

Neck movements should be tested, again to see if they precipitate symptoms, and ears should be examined. Measurement of blood pressure, both lying or sitting and standing should be carried out. If a drop in BP on standing is demonstrated, the patient should be asked whether this produces any symptoms, particularly the dizziness he/she has experienced.

A simple assessment of stance and gait is often useful. Observing the patient standing quietly with feet comfortably apart and with feet together, and with eyes open and closed (with someone nearby in case of instability) provides much information about the integrity of sensory input, and watching him/her walking across the room and turning round is also quite illuminating on occasion. It is rarely necessary to resort to more complicated gait and balance testing.

Investigation

Investigation of dizziness has two elements: simple investigations available to general practitioners, accident departments and non-specialised hospital departments; and more complex and specialised otological (and sometimes neurological) investigations. In the absence of a thorough history and examination, further investigation is difficult, if not impossible, to direct and is unlikely to answer the question about what causes the patient's symptoms. Opinion is divided about how important investigation is in the diagnosis of dizziness, with otologists tending to feel that it is vital, and non-specialists suggesting that investigation should be selective, diagnosis most frequently being made on the basis of a thorough history.

Simple investigations include such things as full blood count, biochemical screen, thyroid function tests and chest radiograph, to look for obvious underlying medical causes for dizziness, particularly if the symptom is vague and non-specific. Anaemia, chronic renal failure or lung neoplasm may explain the dizziness or instability. More sophisticated tests may be indicated in specific situations, such as CT brain scan when history and examination suggest progressive neurological disease.

If the symptom is true vertigo, it may be appropriate to refer for specialised otological investigation. Readers are referred to ENT textbooks for fuller descriptions of tests available. Audiological assessment will demonstrate hearing loss, and the pattern of loss may strengthen (or weaken) a clinical diagnosis. For example, the typical pattern of deafness in Menière's disease is different from the pattern of age-related deafness (presbyacusis). There are a number of patterns of abnormalities on caloric testing (irrigation of the external auditory canal with water at various temperatures and observation of the resulting nystagmus) and electronystagmography (electrical measurement of spontaneous eye movements in response to various stimuli, usually carried out in the dark to remove the suppressive effect of visual fixation) which again can support or refute a clinical diagnosis. Because some of the tests are potentially unpleasant and/or require a substantial degree of cooperation it may not always be appropriate to subject elderly sufferers to them, particularly if the patient is very frail, but in each case a judgement must be made about whether the benefits of a clear diagnosis (which will allow treatment to be more appropriate and prognosis to be more accurate) outweigh the unpleasantness of the investigations.

Treatment

Diagnosis should precede treatment. This is as true for dizziness as it is for any other affliction, but it often seems that the difficulties in reaching a diagnosis of these complaints paralyse doctors. An assumption seems to be made that all dizziness is the same and requires treatment with one of a small range of drugs which are thought to suppress 'dizziness' (i.e. vertigo). Because dizziness is such a common complaint amongst old people, this means that a significant proportion of the elderly population is exposed to such drugs, often inappropriately. In many cases reassurance or non-drug treatment would be more effective, and would avoid the potentially damaging side effects of medication.

If dizziness is considered in the four categories discussed above, treatment options can be more logically considered. Drug treatment may be very effective if the complaint is true vertigo. Syncope and near-syncope may require specific drug or other treatment, and this is considered later in this chapter. The two remaining categories, dysequilibrium and 'other' are rarely helped by the drugs which suppress vertigo, and may in fact be made worse (or even be precipitated) by them. Where these symptoms are a manifestation of an underlying medical condition (anaemia, hypothyroidism, cerebral tumour, etc.) accurate diagnosis and treatment is clearly more appropriate than 'vestibular suppression'. The strong association between non-specific dizziness and psychological morbidity means that antidepressants may be the most appropriate therapy in this group, and a therapeutic trial of an antidepressant may be worth considering. This should be with an appropriate drug at appropriate dosage for long enough to be likely to have an effect, and with reassessment at the end of that time and withdrawal of the drug if there has been no improvement.

It may be helpful to consider briefly the drugs commonly prescribed for 'dizziness', and their role in management of the problem.

Betahistine (Serc)
This is a histamine agonist, which has a dilating effect on the microcirculation of the labyrinth. It may have an effect on regional cerebral blood flow in the vertebrobasilar arterial system. It seems to be effective in Menière's disease and would theoretically be useful in other peripheral vestibular disorders.

Cinnarizine (Stugeron)
This is a calcium channel blocker, therefore having effects on vascular smooth muscle. It is related to cyclizine, and has antihistaminic, sedative and antiemetic effects. It may act to inhibit vasoconstriction produced by other

stimuli but does not directly cause vasodilatation. It would seem, theoretically, to be most useful where the underlying mechanism of dizziness is thought to be vascular insufficiency.

Prochlorperazine (Stemetil)

This is a phenothiazine (a major tranquilliser), which again has sedative and antiemetic effects. In long term use it can lead to parkinsonism, and may in some circumstances precipitate Parkinson's disease (perhaps in those at risk of idiopathic Parkinson's disease because of lower levels of striatal dopamine). It can produce postural hypotension. Its sedative action may be experienced as a feeling of dysequilibrium and will tend to impair alertness, increasing risk of falls. It is rarely an appropriate or useful drug in the management of dizziness except in the acute stages of 'vestibular neuronitis', and at other times usually does more harm than good. It is interesting to speculate that the reason it does sometimes make dizzy old people feel better is when the symptom is a manifestation of an underlying anxiety state. However, there are almost certainly safer ways of treating anxiety in these circumstances than using a phenothiazine.

Non-drug treatment of dizziness

Once people develop vertigo (or the less specific types of dizziness), they often find that movement of the head, neck or body exacerbates the sensations. As a result they may limit movement to try to avoid precipitating symptoms. They tend to hold themselves stiffly, keeping their eyes directed straight ahead, and turning the whole body to look sideways. This produces fatigue, and spasm in the muscles of the neck and shoulders. Symptoms also tend to be worse in the dark or on irregular surfaces, so a sufferer may reduce his/her level of activity to avoid these circumstances. A vicious circle often seems to be produced, with the original symptoms leading to reduced and more tiring activities and loss of confidence, which in turn tends to make symptoms worse. Paradoxically, if sufferers can be encouraged to perform the movement(s) that precipitate the dizziness, compensation often occurs and symptoms diminish. This is the basis on which Cooksey (1945) and Cawthorne (1945) developed a series of exercises for those with acute vestibular failure following surgery for Menière's disease and sufferers of post-concussional vertigo. The technique is a graded series of exercises, starting with movements of the eyes only, progressing through movements of head and neck with eyes open and closed, to movements of the whole body.

Balance retraining (see Chapter 7) works on a similar principle and is frequently also appropriate for those with dizziness. These sorts of exercises are also helpful in those with non-specific dizziness due to cervical spondylosis. Such patients have often been given cervical collars in the mistaken belief that their symptoms are due to 'vertebrobasilar insufficiency' caused by nipping of the vertebral arteries by cervical osteophytes, and that reducing neck movements will prevent this. Cervical collars will further limit the proprioceptive input from cervical mechanoreceptors, tending to make dizziness worse, whereas Cooksey–Cawthorne exercises and balance retraining may help by increasing proprioceptive input and improving confidence.

Psychological aspects of dizziness

The relationship between somatic and psychological symptoms is often close, and with any illness the psychological reactions both to illness generally and to the specific symptoms of the disease affect the way in which the disease presents, progresses and responds to treatment. Vertigo, syncope and dysequilibrium frequently provoke emotional distress, partly perhaps because they are associated with a feeling of loss of control. Because the general public's commonest exposure to (and experience of) unsteadiness is in the context of alcoholic intoxication, people who are unsteady fear that they will be thought to be drunk, and this can be particularly upsetting to older people of temperate habit.

This group of symptoms provides a good example of the close interrelationship between soma and psyche. They seem to be particularly likely to produce psychological responses (somatopsychic) but may be a purely psychological problem presenting with physical symptoms (psychosomatic). More commonly the problem is somewhere on the continuum between the purely somatic and the purely psychological.

The relationship between dizziness and psychological symptoms has been studied to a limited extent. Subjects with dizziness have been shown in a number of studies to be more functionally disabled (Sixt and Landahl, 1987; Sloane et al., 1989; Downton and Andrews, 1990), but in addition, there has been shown to be a particularly strong relationship with anxiety and depression, with these two factors being the strongest 'predictors' of dizziness on discriminant analysis (Downton and Andrews, 1990). Dizziness is strongly associated with fear of falling, but only weakly associated with having actually fallen in the previous 12 months. It has been suggested that there are two categories of dizzy patients, those with anxiety, depression and somatization and those with neurosensory or cardiovascular problems (Sloane et al., 1989). A questionnaire to ascertain the impact of dizziness on sufferers (The Dizziness Handicap Inventory) has been devised, including questions about physical, functional and emotional aspects of dizziness and unsteadiness (Jacobson and Newman, 1990). Scores for the functional and emotional elements increased significantly with frequency of dizziness episodes.

A study of elderly psychiatric patients found a high incidence of symptoms of dizziness (though it was only slightly higher than the general population of that age). Although physical disease and drugs taken were important causes of dizziness (often mediated through postural hypotension) these factors did not fully explain the high incidence of such symptoms, supporting the suggestion that psychological dysfunction is associated with dizziness (Davie et al., 1981). Dizziness may be one of the symptoms of agoraphobia (Orma and Koskenoja, 1957a).

These studies do not tell us whether the dizziness caused the psychological distress or vice versa, and it is likely that causation occurs in both directions. What they do indicate is the degree to which the two are related, which means that anyone attempting to manage patients with dizziness needs to consider psychological state, both in diagnosis and treatment.

Case report

An 80 year-old woman was admitted to hospital following a fall resulting in a soft tissue injury to her leg. This settled with analgesia and she was gradually mobilised. She had previously been fit and well, but reported a number of falls in the previous few months, which appeared to be due to simple trips. She had become anxious because of the falls and had lost her confidence. She complained of a continuous sensation of dizziness which she was unable to describe more specifically on further questioning. Staff on the ward felt she was depressed, and she scored highly on a geriatric depression scale. She was treated with a tricyclic antidepressant, and over the next month became less anxious and her symptoms of dizziness disappeared.

Syncope

The definition of syncope is a sudden, brief loss of consciousness due to transient global impairment of cerebral circulation, usually occurring in the absence of organic brain disease or cerebrovascular disease, with spontaneous recovery (Ormerod, 1984). It has a number of synonyms (both medical and lay), including faint, loss of consciousness, seizure, collapse, blackout, 'stroke', unresponsiveness, passing out, and so on, and like dizziness and its synonyms, these terms may not mean the same to doctors as they do to patients. The typical clinical picture is of an episode with an onset that is sudden, or developing over a few seconds, with blurring of vision or darkening of visual field, and associated with manifestations of autonomic activity such as cold extremities, sweating and nausea. However, other symptom patterns may be covered by the term, and there is an overlap between syncope, near syncope and 'dizziness' as discussed above.

How common is syncope?

There have been no studies specifically looking at the frequency of syncope in representative elderly populations, though studies of young people suggest that the symptom is a very common one. For all age groups syncope is reported to account for 1–3 per cent of attendances at accident and emergency departments and 3–6 per cent of hospital admissions (Anonymous, 1991).

A North American screening survey, looking at a wide range of symptoms amongst those over 65 found that about 6 per cent of men and women reported episodes of blacking out, and 8.3 per cent of women and 6.5 per cent of men reported sensations of fainting or floating (Hale et al., 1986). The frequency with which such symptoms were reported increased with increasing age. In the Newcastle community study, a higher proportion, 26 per cent, of those aged 65 and over said they had suffered faints or blackouts (Evans, 1990). In a group of institutionalised elderly people, there was a yearly incidence of syncope of 6 per cent, and a 10-year prevalence of 23 per cent. Over two years there was a recurrence rate of 30 per cent (Lipsitz et al., 1985).

Patients with syncope often present to casualty departments, but no figures are available about how commonly this occurs. In a study of people aged 65 and over presenting to an Accident and Emergency Department with falls, 12 per cent complained of loss of consciousness, though in another 58 per cent it was not known or not stated whether loss of consciousness had occurred (Paramsothy and Downton, 1992). A study of patients of all ages found that 3 per cent of attenders at an emergency room were seen for complaints that might be associated with loss of consciousness (Day et al., 1982). When those with known seizure disorder and head trauma were excluded, less than 1 per cent had syncope.

Studies looking at elderly subjects with syncope presenting to medical attention suggest that a cause is identified in approximately 60–70 per cent (Lipsitz et al., 1985; Kapoor et al., 1986a). Mortality rate following syncope is probably not increased in the elderly compared to an age-matched population (Lipsitz et al., 1985), though a cardiovascular cause does seem to lead to an increased mortality (Kapoor et al., 1986a; Day et al., 1982). A fall resulting from syncope seems to be more likely to lead to injury, particularly severe injury such as fractures, than falls without loss of consciousness (Kapoor et al., 1986a).

Epidemiological studies of falls and fractures give some information about the frequency with which these events arise from dizziness and syncope, though differences in terminology mean that it is not possible to compare studies directly. The New Zealand community study (Campbell et al., 1981) reported that 6 per cent of falls were caused by 'drop attack or syncopal vertebrobasilar insufficiency' and 3 per cent by 'postural hypotension'. In the Newcastle study (Prudham and Evans, 1981) 6 per cent of falls resulted from 'dizziness or vertigo' and 4 per cent from loss of consciousness. Their study also reported that 33 per cent of fallers and 24 per cent of non-fallers reported faints or blackouts at some time. In the Nottingham study (Blake et al., 1988), 8 per cent of falls followed 'dizziness' and 6 per cent 'blackout'.

A prospective, community based study of people over 70 in New Zealand, (Campbell et al., 1989) found that 24 out of 268 falls were associated with loss of consciousness, in four of which a single cause was identified (epilepsy in two, aortic stenosis and Stokes–Adams attacks in one each), and in the remaining 20 a combination of causes was thought to be responsible.

Causes of syncope

Syncope is in some ways easier than dizziness to assess and characterise because it is a much more clearly defined entity than dizziness and it is also more objective. If a witness is present it is usually abundantly clear that consciousness has been lost. However, in the absence of a witness, an elderly person may sometimes be uncertain whether loss of consciousness has occurred.

Because of the additive effects of age-related physiological changes and disease on cerebral oxygen delivery, many elderly are near the critical threshold of cerebral oxygenation for central nervous system dysfunction (Lipsitz, 1983). Common conditions such as congestive heart failure, anaemia, cerebrovascular disease and chronic lung disease can all reduce blood oxygen content and/or cerebral blood flow. In these circumstances it is easy to see why an apparently trivial additional stress may result in loss of consciousness, and why the elderly are more likely to black out when they become acutely ill than young people.

There are only a limited number of mechanisms by which loss of consciousness can be produced:

1. impaired circulation of blood to the brain;

2. impaired cerebral metabolism;

3. alteration in electrical activity within the brain.

These are the 'final common pathways' of syncope, but for clinical management it is perhaps more helpful to think of the main types of problems that give rise to syncope (Table 6.4). There is clearly some overlap (Fig. 6.3), particularly between cardiovascular causes and hypotension, in that the mechanism by which cardiovascular causes lead to syncope is through hypotension. Problems in one group may lead to others in another group. For example, a cardiac arrhythmia or postural hypotension may be followed by an anoxic fit. This classification is not exhaustive, but covers most of the important causes. Some of the causes of syncope listed here are discussed in more detail in Chapter 5.

The 'specific' types of syncope (cough, micturition, defecation and swallow syncope) are probably syndromes with multiple aetiologies (Kapoor et al., 1985; 1986b) rather than clear-cut pathophysiological conditions. The mechanisms of syncope in these cases includes the Valsalva manoeuvre whilst straining, vagal stimulation by a full bladder, reflex vasodilatation by bladder

Table 6.4 Causes of syncope.

Cardiovascular	Arrhythmias	Bradyarrhythmias
		Tacharrhythmias
		Sick sinus syndrome
	Transient myocardial dysfunction	Ischaemia
		Aortic stenosis
		HOCM
Hypotension	Vasovagal	
	Specific types	Cough syncope
		Micturition syncope
		Defaecation syncope
		Swallow syncope
	Postural hypotension	Autonomic neuropathy
		Drug related
		Volume depletion
Hypoglycaemia	Drug induced	Oral hypoglycaemics
		Insulin
	Spontaneous	Reactive
		Insulinoma
		Liver disease
		Addisons disease
		Malignant disease
Epilepsy		
Other	Hypocalcaemia	
	Hyperventilation	

emptying and decline in reflex cardio-acceleration with cough (Lipsitz, 1983). It is often possible to limit the symptoms of such syndromes by simple interventions (such as advising elderly men with micturition syncope to urinate sitting down), therefore a clear clinical diagnosis can be helpful in management.

Studies of syncope in adults of all ages suggest that the commonest cause is a vasovagal faint. Of adults presenting to an emergency room with transient loss of consciousness, 40 per cent had suffered a vasovagal attack (this group

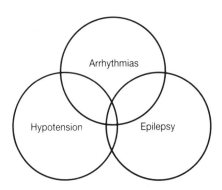

Fig. 6.3   Overlap of factors giving rise to loss of consciousness

included those with an orthostatic faint), 29 per cent had had seizures, small percentages had other CNS causes, cardiac causes and drug and metabolic causes, and 13 per cent did not have a clear diagnosis (Day et al., 1982). A comparison of elderly and younger patients with syncope (accrued from emergency room attenders, inpatients and outpatients) found that a cardiovascular cause was significantly commoner in the elderly group, with vasovagal faint being much less common (Kapoor et al., 1986a).

Assessment of syncope

The sensible assessment and investigation of syncope is hampered by the multiplicity of conditions that can cause loss of consciousness and by the frequency with which the blackout is unwitnessed in the elderly. However, studies have shown that the cause of the attack can be determined with a fair degree of confidence from a thorough history and examination in many people with syncope, though the proportion is less in the elderly (about 40 per cent) than in adults generally (about 85 per cent) (Day et al., 1982; Kapoor et al., 1986a). History therefore is the cornerstone of diagnosis.

History

If possible a history should be obtained from a witness as well as the patient, as the patient will be unable to describe events during the period of unconsciousness. Important factors to ascertain include the duration of the attack, any obvious trigger activities or events, and the speed of onset and recovery. Pre-syncopal activity will often give important clues: micturition (particularly at night in males with prostatic hypertrophy), defecation, or a coughing fit are obvious diagnostic pointers; use of one or both arms prior to the attack may indicate subclavian steal; postural changes suggests orthostatic hypotension; neck movement raises the possibility of vertebrobasilar insufficiency (which is, however, somewhat over-diagnosed); and effort suggests a cardiac cause, as does chest pain or palpitations preceding the blackout. A description of the appearance of the patient during and after the attack can be helpful. The deathly pallor during, and red flush after a Stokes–Adams attack are characteristic, but the presence of jerking of limbs and urinary incontinence during the attack do not prove epilepsy since syncope of other types may be followed by an anoxic fit. Those who have had a fit tend to take longer to come round, and frequently have a post-ictal headache and confusion. A post-ictal confusional state can be very prolonged, sometimes lasting several days, even if mental function is normal between attacks, though sufferers with chronic confusional states tend to take longer to return to normal.

A more general history should also be taken and may reveal symptoms suggesting underlying neurological, cardiac or respiratory disease. A drug history should not be forgotten, and should include over-the-counter medications as well as prescribed drugs.

Examination

This should be aimed particularly at discovering abnormal neurological signs and evidence of cardiovascular disease, such as vascular bruits, absent pulses and cardiac murmurs. Blood pressure should be measured in the lying or sitting and standing position to look for a postural drop in blood pressure and symptoms of dizziness or lightheadedness. The presence of a postural drop without symptoms is less helpful than the presence of symptoms of postural dizziness, with or without a drop in blood pressure. Orthostatic hypotension is quite common in the asymptomatic elderly (Caird et al., 1973) in whom cerebral autoregulation is presumably capable of maintaining cerebral blood flow despite the drop in systemic blood pressure.

There is now some evidence that carotid sinus hypersensitivity is a significant cause of syncope in the elderly (Kenny and Traynor, 1991). Testing for such hypersensitivity in a standardised way, by carotid sinus massage for six seconds on each side (with a minimum interval of one minute between sides), should be part of the assessment of unexplained syncope. The test is positive if stimulation produces asystole of three seconds or more, or a fall in systolic pressure of greater than 50 mmHg. It is sensible to have equipment for cardiac resuscitation at hand during such testing.

If the presentation of syncope is acute then the possibility of acute medical and surgical emergencies such as myocardial infarction, pulmonary embolus, aortic dissection, gastrointestinal haemorrhage and acute abdominal disasters should be considered. A general examination should always be carried out.

Investigation

To some extent this should be guided by the findings from history and examination. In the absence of clear clues to aetiology it is sensible to carry out full blood count, biochemical screen (including urea, electrolytes, creatinine and blood sugar), chest X-ray and ECG. As an important differential diagnosis is a cardiac arrhythmia a 24-hour ECG is often worth performing, though the high prevalence of cardiac arrhythmias and the low correlation between symptoms and the presence of arrhythmias in the elderly sometimes makes interpretation difficult. In addition, where symptoms are intermittent, the likelihood of 'catching' an arrhythmia may not be high. The place of electroencephalogram (EEG) is less clear, since a normal EEG does not exclude epilepsy and an abnormal one does not prove its presence.

In specific situations more complex tests may be helpful, such as CT brain scanning, echocardiogram, electrophysiological tests, glucose tolerance tests, and so on, but in the majority of cases, these sorts of invasive (and often expensive) investigations do not improve diagnostic yield (Kapoor et al.,

1982). Where it is not possible to come to a definitive diagnosis, a therapeutic trial, usually of anticonvulsants or antiarrhythmics, is sometimes justified, though again may be difficult to interpret in those with long gaps between episodes. Doing nothing, observing events and reassessing the patient intermittently are often the most useful procedures to follow, and at least avoid adding iatrogenic disease to the underlying disorder.

Management

This is theoretically straightforward, but in practice the difficulties in diagnosis lead to difficulties in management. Where a clear diagnosis is made, treatment of the underlying cause should solve the problem, but the fact that drug treatment may be toxic should be remembered. Antiarrhythmics in particular have many possible problems, not least a potential for proarrhythmic action (Velebit et al., 1982).

Where postural hypotension is the cause, and underlying reasons such as inappropriate drug treatment or fluid depletion have been dealt with as far as possible, a number of techniques can be tried. Compression stockings often help, but are difficult for frail elderly people to put on and take off without assistance. Propping up the head of the bed, so that the sufferer is never completely flat, sometimes helps, as does exercising the arms and legs before getting up. Occasionally it is necessary to try treatment with mineralocorticoids, though side effects are common.

Because syncope in the elderly is commonly multifactorial, attention to general health is important. Simple interventions such as avoidance of unnecessary medication, maintenance of adequate fluid intake and care when getting up from bed or chair may be more useful than specific interventions.

Case report

A home visit was requested to assess an 84 year-old man, who was reported to have congestive heart failure, for which he had been prescribed a loop diuretic, though his GP felt that he did not take his medication regularly. He had had a number of falls over the preceding five days, resulting in a minor head injury. He was normally fairly well and active, and usually looked after his disabled wife and handicapped daughter. On examination he had no clinical evidence of cardiac failure, but was hypotensive. His sitting blood pressure was 110/70, and standing blood pressure was unrecordable. Standing up resulted in a faint. Biochemical screen was normal apart from a mildly raised urea. His diuretic was stopped, and over the next few days his postural hypotension resolved and his urea returned to normal.

References

Anonymous (1991). Explaining syncope (Editorial). *Lancet*. **338**: 353–354.

Baloh, R.W., Honrubia, V. and Jacobson, K. (1987). Benign positional vertigo: clinical and oculographic features in 240 cases. *Neurology*. **37:** 371–378.
Baloh, R.W., Sloane, P.D. and Honrubia, V. (1989). Quantitative vestibular function testing in elderly patients with dizziness. *Ear Nose Throat J*. **68:** 935–939.
Belal, A. and Glorig, A. (1986). Disequilibrium of aging (presbyastasis). *J Laryngol Otol*. **100:** 1037–1041.
Blake, A.J., Morgan, K., Bendall, M.J., Dallosso, H., Ebrahim, S.B.J., Arie, T.H.D., Fentem, P.H. and Bassey, E.J. (1988). Falls by elderly people at home: prevalence and associated factors. *Age Ageing*. **17:** 365–372.
Caird, F.I., Andrews, G.R. and Kennedy, R.D. (1973). Effect of posture on blood pressure in the elderly. *Br Heart J*. **35:** 527–530.
Campbell, A.J., Borrie, M.J. and Spears, G.F. (1989). Risk factors for falls in a community-based prospective study of people 70 years and older. *J Gerontol*. **44:** M112–M117.
Campbell, A.J., Reinken, J., Allan, B.C. and Martinez, G.S. (1981). Falls in old age: a study of frequency and related clinical factors. *Age Ageing*. **10:** 264–270.
Cawthorne, T. (1945). Vestibular injuries. *Proc Roy Soc Med*. **39:** 270–273.
Cooksey, F.S. (1945). Rehabilitation in vestibular injuries. *Proc Roy Soc Med*. **39:** 273–278.
Davie, J.W., Blumenthal, M.D. and Robinson-Hawkins, S. (1981). A model of risk of falling for psychogeriatric patients. *Arch Gen Psych*. **38:** 463–467.
Day, S.C., Cook, E.F., Funkenstein, H. and Goldman, L. (1982). Evaluation and outcome of emergency room patients with transient loss of consciousness. *Am J Med*. **73:** 15–23.
Downton, J.H. and Andrews, K. (1990). Postural disturbance and psychological symptoms amongst elderly people living at home. *Int J Geriatr Psychiatry*. **5:** 93–98.
Drachmann, D.A. and Hart, C.W. (1972). An approach to the dizzy patient. *Neurology*. **22:** 323–334.
Droller, H. (1955). Falls among elderly people living at home. *Geriatrics*. **10:** 239–244.
Evans, J.G. (1990). Transient neurological dysfunction and risk of stroke in an elderly English population: the different significance of vertigo and non-rotatory dizziness. *Age Ageing*. **19:** 43–49.
Goodwin, J.S. and Regan, M. (1982). Cognitive dysfunction associated with naproxen and ibuprofen in the elderly. *Arthr Rheum*. **25:** 1013–1014.
Hale, W.E., Perkins, L.L., May, F.E., Marks, R.G. and Stewart, R.B. (1986). Symptom prevalence in the elderly. An evaluation of age, sex, disease and medication use. *J Am Geriatr Soc*. **34:** 333–340.
Hale, W.E., Stewart, R.B. and Marks, R.G. (1984). Central nervous system symptoms of elderly subjects using antihypertensive drugs. *J Am Geriatr Soc*. **32:** 5–10.
Jacobson, G.P. and Newman, C.W. (1990). The development of the Dizziness Handicap Inventory. *Arch Otolaryngol Head Neck Surg*. **116:** 424–427.
Kapoor, W., Snustad, D., Peterson, J., Wieand, H.S., Cha, R. and Karpf, M. (1986a). Syncope in the elderly. *Am J Med*. **80:** 419–427.
Kapoor, W.N., Karpf, M., Maher, Y., Miller, R.A. and Levey, G.S. (1982). Syncope of unknown origin. The need for a more cost effective approach to its diagnostic evaluation. *JAMA*. **247:** 2687–2691.
Kapoor, W.N., Peterson, J.R. and Karpf, M. (1985). Micturition syncope. A reappraisal. *JAMA*. **253:** 796–798.
Kapoor, W.N., Peterson, J.R. and Karpf, M. (1986b). Defecation syncope. A symptom with multiple etiologies. *Arch Intern Med*. **146:** 2377–2379.
Kenny, R.A. and Traynor, G. (1991). Carotid sinus syndrome – clinical characteristics in elderly patients. *Age Ageing*. **20:** 449–454.
Lipsitz, L.A. (1983). Syncope in the elderly. *Ann Intern Med*. **99:** 92–105.

Lipsitz, L.A., Wei, J.Y. and Rowe, J.W. (1985). Syncope in an elderly institutionalised population: prevalence, incidence and associated risk. *Q J Med*. **55:** 45–54.

Lucht, U. (1971). A prospective study of accidental falls and resulting injuries in the home among elderly people. *Acta Socio-Med Scand*. **3:** 105–120.

Orma, E.J. and Koskenoja, M. (1957a). Dizziness attacks and continuous dizziness in the aged. *Geriatrics*. **12:** 92–100.

Orma, E.J. and Koskenoja, M. (1957b). Postural dizziness in the aged. *Geriatrics*. **12:** 49–59.

Ormerod, A.D. (1984). Syncope. (Clinical Algorithms). *Br Med J*. **288:** 1219–1222.

Overstall, P.W., Hazell, J.W.P. and Johnson, A.L. (1981). Vertigo in the elderly. *Age Ageing*. **10:** 105–109.

Paramsothy, V. and Downton, J.H. (1992). Elderly people presenting to Accident and Emergency departments with falls. (Manuscript in preparation.)

Prudham, D. and Evans, J.G. (1981). Factors associated with falls in the elderly: a community study. *Age Ageing*. **10:** 141–146.

Sheldon, J.H. (1948). *The Social Medicine of Old Age. Report of an inquiry in Wolverhampton*. London, Oxford University Press.

Sixt, E. and Landahl, S. (1987). Postural disturbances in a 75 year old population. I. Prevalence and functional consequences. *Age Ageing*. **16:** 393–398.

Sloane, P., Blazer, D. and George, L.K. (1989). Dizziness in an community elderly population. *J Am Geriatr Soc*. **37:** 101–108.

Sloane, P.D. (1989). Dizziness in primary care. Results from the National Ambulatory Medical Care Survey. *J Fam Pract*. **29:** 33–38.

Sloane, P.D. and Baloh, R.W. (1989). Persistent dizziness in geriatric patients. *J Am Geriatrics Soc*. **37:** 1031–1038.

Spitzer, J.B. (1990). An evaluation of the relationship among electronystagmographic, audiologic, and self-report descriptors of dizziness. *Eur Arch Otorhinolaryngol*. **247:** 114–118.

Velebit, V., Podrid, P., Lown, B., Cohen, B.H. and Graboys, T.B. (1982). Aggravation and provocation of ventricular arrhythmias by antiarrhythmic drugs. *Circulation*. **65:** 886–894.

Chapter 7

Clinical management of fallers

There is little systematic information about how the problems of elderly fallers are managed in the various sections of the hospital and community services. A proportion of falls are not reported to medical attention, and of those that are, a further proportion do not require, or do not receive, any further medical attention. It is not clear, however, how large these proportions are, nor how appropriate is the management that they receive. There is a suggestion from preliminary studies that multidisciplinary assessment (including social and environmental assessment) and involvement of remedial therapists may benefit elderly fallers (Burley, 1983; Wolf-Klein et al., 1988), but at present there is no definitive evidence. It seems likely, however, that a more thoughtful, uniform and coordinated approach to the management of falls and fallers would have clinical and economic advantages.

There are two main elements to the management of falls. First, there is the assessment and management of the faller once a fall has occurred, and secondly, there is general evaluation of both elderly person and environment to look for (alterable) factors increasing risk of falls and injury. Assessment of fallers, particularly at the time of, or shortly after the fall, is obviously necessary to detect any injury, but it is also often possible to pick up potentially treatable causes or predisposing factors for falls.

Not all elderly fallers have complicated problems. A proportion have suffered straightforward falls such as might happen at any age. For these reasons, a system of 'triage' should be used, to separate those who can safely be reassured and discharged from those who need further attention, either because of injuries, or because their fall is a marker of a significant medical problem.

The essential question to try to answer is: why did this particular person fall at this particular time in this particular place? This implies that there are internal, external (environmental), and situational factors which may be fixed but are more likely to be variable with time. Although there is an 'environmental' element to all falls, this does not mean that adapting the environment will stop falls occurring; merely that for an individual with a particular

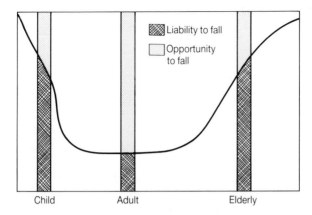

Fig. 7.1 Contribution of liability to fall and opportunity to fall at different ages

intrinsic degree of 'fall-proneness', external and situational factors affect the likelihood of a fall now rather than an hour ago or an hour hence. For a fall to occur, there must be an 'opportunity' as well as a 'liability' to fall. However unsteady people are, they cannot fall if they have no opportunity to fall. The relative contributions of 'liability' and 'opportunity' vary at different ages (Fig. 7.1) and contribute to the different rates of falling with age. They also vary in a less predictable way with time, and someone with a particular liability to fall today may have a smaller or larger liability tomorrow because of a change in health, medication, mental state or environment. Almost any medical condition may increase an elderly person's risk of falling; conversely, not everyone with a particular problem suffers falls, nor does someone with the problem fall all the time. A proportion of falls (at any age) occurs for predominantly 'external' reasons – so-called 'trips' or 'slips'. Changes with ageing may make trips or slips more likely because of changes in gait, and they may make falls more likely if trips or slips occur because of slowed reactions and impaired righting reflexes.

Because falls are so common, the problem of dealing with elderly people who have fallen is a frequent and widespread one, and a faller may present to someone who is aware of the particular health problems of the elderly or to someone who does not see these as his/her concern. Elderly people who have suffered a fall present in a number of different ways. They may present acutely ('I've just fallen'), usually to their general practitioner or to an Accident and Emergency Department, or they may present non-acutely, either because of a single fall or with recurrent falling ('I've had lots of falls', 'I keep falling'). Their carers may ask for help because of recurrent, minor falls, or a history of falls may become apparent during an assessment for other medical or social problems. Management may need to be different in these different circumstances, though many aspects are common to all these situations. In many ways, the procedure that needs to be followed is much the same wherever the faller presents. However, the emphasis differs, and it is therefore worth considering the specific elements of relevance in particular situations.

General principles of management of falls

Clearly, the first priority is to identify and deal with any injury sustained. Once this has been done and the patient's condition is stabilised, the question of what caused the fall can be addressed.

There is always a reason why someone falls. It is usually possible to determine at least some of the factors that have caused the fall, and it is often possible to do something about some or all of them to reduce the risk of further falls (Rubenstein et al., 1988). In order to do this it is however necessary to actually ask about what happened, and to ask in a way which will allow the elderly person to provide useful information about what has happened. Without careful enquiry the faller may not necessarily be able to organise his/her description into something that the health professional can interpret, and the scene will be set for misunderstandings and potentially mistaken assumptions about what is going on.

History

What should you ask an elderly person who has had a fall? A general question such as 'why did you fall?' or 'what caused your fall?' may not provide much helpful information, though people who have had a straightforward trip or slip may be able to describe the circumstances of their fall in response to such questions. A note of caution here – there is often an element of rationalisation. 'I fell. People fall because they trip. Therefore I must have tripped.' If the patient says 'I *must have* tripped' then it is quite likely that he/she did not trip. If, however, the faller is able to describe clearly the cause of the fall and the circumstances leading up to it (for example tripping over uneven paving stones, slipping on a patch of ice, etc.) then the fall can more confidently be ascribed to a trip or slip. Another caution is that ill-health may mean that an elderly person is more likely to trip, as well as suffer a 'non-trip' fall, and it is therefore important that the possibility of an underlying illness is considered, even if the fall was clearly due to a simple trip.

If the fall is of a 'non-specific' or 'non-trip' type, it must then be considered whether the fall was the presenting feature of an acute illness of any type. If this does not seem to be the case, then the wide range of potential causative or contributory factors needs to be considered.

More useful questions than 'what happened' are:

What were you doing at the time of your fall (e.g. walking, standing still, getting up from a chair, bending over, turning the head)?

What were you doing immediately before your fall?

Were you feeling quite well before you fell?

Did you notice any symptoms (e.g. dizziness, palpitation, chest pain, visual disturbance) prior to, or following, your fall?

Did you black out or lose consciousness when you fell?

Did you feel as if you were going to black out when you fell?

How did you feel after your fall?

How long did it take you to recover?

Symptoms such as 'dizziness' or 'palpitations' need to be carefully defined, as they may describe a number of different sensations (see Chapter 6). Loss of consciousness also needs to be carefully considered, as not everyone uses 'black out' and 'loss of consciousness' as synonyms. A careful balance needs to be struck between allowing the faller to describe the events in his/her own words and the judicious use of leading questions, to clarify sensations which to the faller may have been mystifying and frightening.

Where the complaint is that 'I've had lots of falls', there are a few further questions that may be helpful in clarifying the situation. Have the falls all been similar and/or occurred in similar circumstances? If so this suggests a single cause, or a limited number of mechanisms underlying the falls, and a description of a typical fall should be obtained. If there is no pattern to the falls, it is more likely that there are a number of underlying problems.

The description of the fall that is obtained from the faller may be very vague or non-existent, and in the absence of a witness, it is often difficult to know how much reliance to place upon it, particularly if there is any cognitive impairment. If a witness is available, particularly if it is possible to interview him/her shortly after the fall, as much information as possible should be obtained about the circumstances of the fall, the appearance of the faller, whether there was any loss of consciousness, how the faller seemed after the fall, and whether there have been previous similar episodes. Any information about how the faller behaved before and after the event is also useful.

An enquiry as to the faller's normal functional status is helpful. The likely causes of a fall in someone who is normally poorly mobile and very dependent may well be different from those in a healthy, independent, elderly person. In the frail elderly there are likely to be a number of conditions that increase the risk of falling, and it can sometimes be difficult to know which is the prime cause. In the fit elderly it is more likely that there is a single cause. Questions about how steady the faller is on his/her feet normally may be useful, and use of mobility aids, such as sticks or walking frames, should be ascertained.

Because of the wide range of potential causes of falls, and the fact that factors may interact to produce an increased risk of falling, a thorough medical history is usually necessary. Drug treatment has been clearly implicated in causing some falls, and in increasing risk of falling, so medication, both prescribed and over-the-counter, must be reviewed. Alcohol intake should also be considered, and information may need to be obtained from relatives or carers about level of alcohol consumption as those with a serious drink problem may not admit to their actual intake.

An enquiry about home circumstances, to identify environmental risks, is useful, and in some circumstances needs to be supplemented by a visit to the faller's home.

Examination

In many cases a full medical examination is appropriate, particularly if the fall seems to be due to acute illness, which may be in any system of the body. It is also often appropriate in the assessment of someone having recurrent falls, when again the problem or problems may be in any body system. The history may indicate specific areas of examination, for example if the fall was associated with dizziness (see Chapter 6).

There are a number of specific factors which may be useful in the examination of someone who has fallen. A cardiovascular examination, including pulse rate and rhythm and supine and standing blood pressure, should be carried out. Whilst looking for orthostatic hypotension the faller should be asked about whether there is any postural dizziness or lightheadedness, which may be present despite no measurable drop in blood pressure on standing. Where there is a strong suspicion from the history that postural hypotension is the cause of the falls, but no drop is measured initially, it is worth continuing measurement of blood pressure for some time, as there may be a later drop in pressure. Carotid sinus massage (carried out with facilities for resuscitation at hand) may demonstrate evidence of carotid sinus hypersensitivity, of particular relevance if falls are associated with syncope or near-syncope. Cognitive function should be assessed, using as a screening test one of the various ten or twelve question Mental Status Questionnaires (Fig. 7.2). It is worth doing an MSQ on every faller, as a good 'social cover' may hide substantial cognitive impairment, which if present means that information from the history may need to be corroborated.

A neurological examination is usually worthwhile, though it may not identify functional mobility problems (Tinetti and Ginter, 1988). Particular areas meriting attention include visual acuity and visual fields, proximal muscle power, and symmetry of muscle power and reflexes, looking for evidence of cerebrovascular disease or cervical myelopathy. The possibility of Parkinson's disease should be considered, though clear signs may not always be present, as loss of postural reflexes may be the first manifestation of the disease. If there is a possibility of peripheral neuropathy, sensory assessment may be useful, though it is often difficult, especially in the frail elderly. Neck movements should be assessed, to see whether they precipitate dizziness or signs of brainstem vascular insufficiency. Subjects with limited neck movements due to cervical spondylosis may complain of feelings of unsteadiness because of impairment of somatosensory input from cervical spine mecha-

CAPE Information/orientation questionnaire. (*Source*: Pattie and Gilleard, 1975.)		
Name	Address	Colour of British flag
Age	City	Day
Date of birth	Prime Minister	Month
Place	US President	Year
Abbreviated Mental Test Score (*Source*: Qureshi and Hodkinson, 1974)		
Age		
Time (to nearest hour)		
Address for recall at end of test – this should be repeated by the patient to ensure it has been correctly heard: 42 West Street		
Year		
Name of institution or place		
Recognition of two persons (doctor, nurse, etc.)		
Date of Birth (day and month sufficient)		
Year of First World War		
Name of present Monarch		
Count backwards 20–1		

Fig. 7.2   Mental status questionnaires

noreceptors, and these sensations may be precipitated by neck movements. If the faller complains of vertigo, specific examination of the vestibular system may be helpful (see Chapter 6).

Orthopaedic problems which may be relevant are mainly in the lower limbs. In particular the presence of foot deformities should be sought, as even such apparently trivial problems as hallux valgus may contribute to difficulty in walking. Knee joint deformities, such as hyperextension or fixed flexion deformities can interfere with safe mobility, and lateral stability should be determined. The feet should be inspected to reveal 'minor' problems such as long toenails or corns and callosities which may interfere with or cause pain on walking. Finally, a simple assessment of gait and mobility such as the 'Get up and go test' (asking the subject to stand up from a chair, walk across the room, turn round, walk back to the chair and sit down again) (Mathias et al., 1986), or other similar tests should be carried out (Tinetti, 1986).

Investigation

This will depend very much on the particular circumstances of the falls and on which conditions are felt to be causative or contributory. The investigation of elderly fallers with dizziness or syncope has been discussed in Chapter 6. There is a fairly strong argument for doing a number of simple screening investigations on most elderly fallers, because of the tendency of elderly people not to produce the standard, 'textbook', symptoms and signs when ill, and the well-recognised diagnostic difficulties of ill-health in older people. Such investigations should probably include a full blood count, biochemical screen (preferably including creatinine and calcium as well as urea and electrolytes) and thyroid function tests. In fallers presenting acutely a chest X-ray and ECG are usually appropriate.

In those whose symptoms suggest cardiac arrhythmias 24-hour Holter monitoring is often carried out. Interpretation is complicated by the frequency of asymptomatic arrhythmias in healthy elderly, and the tendency for symptoms to disappear whilst the monitor is in place! If there is a strong clinical suspicion that cardiac arrhythmias are occurring, monitoring may need to be repeated several (and sometimes many) times, or Cardiomemo equipment (which allows monitoring to be instigated by the sufferer to 'catch' the arrhythmia) may be helpful. Occurrence of the symptoms without rhythm disturbance whilst the monitor is in place may also allow exclusion of cardiac arrhythmia as a cause.

Simple observation of the faller in situations of risk may be helpful in identifying problems with mobility, but more complex assessment of postural control using equipment in a gait laboratory is not usually of much help in the clinical management of fallers, though it has allowed investigators to identify some of the factors which predispose the elderly to falling.

Case report

An 87 year-old man was transferred to a geriatric ward for rehabilitation following a fractured neck of femur. On assessment he was generally well, but was noted to have a slow pulse and postural hypotension. Electrocardiogram revealed Mobitz Type II atrioventricular block. Review of previous admissions to hospital following repeated falls, some associated with loss of consciousness, showed that he had intermittently had first and second degree heart block noted on ECGs carried out in hospital. Twenty-four hour ECG recording demonstrated intermittent complete heart block. He was transferred for permanent cardiac pacing, and made a good recovery from that and his fracture. He had no further falls over the next year.

Treatment

Once any injury has been dealt with, treatment of a faller will be dictated by the assessment of the cause of the fall. Identification of specific medical factors as probable causes should lead to those factors being improved as far as possible by appropriate intervention, such as stopping an offending drug or altering type of medication. In situations where the cause seems predominantly external, environmental assessment by an occupational therapist may be useful to identify potential risks, though people are often reluctant to make adaptations to their surroundings. It is impossible to get rid of all risks, and attempts to do so may lead to unacceptable restrictions of the autonomy of elderly people.

In the frail elderly with multiple medical and functional problems there is often a defeatist feeling that there are so many problems that nothing can be done. In fact small adjustments in medication, physical activity or mental state may mean the difference between institutionalisation and independence, and it is always worthwhile looking for small treatable elements in larger, more intractable problems. Optimisation of sensory abilities, in particular, may improve functional abilities and morale, and may be as simple as providing new glasses or removing impacted wax from the ears.

Gait assessment and retraining by a physiotherapist may be helpful. The only reported study of physiotherapy for fallers failed to show a clear benefit (Obonyo et al., 1983), but the comparison in that study was between a short and a long period of physiotherapy, so that the value of physiotherapy has not been compared with no treatment. Improving general fitness and mobility would seem to be useful in reducing further falls, in that those who are less fit or have muscle weakness seem more prone to fall and to suffer injury if they do fall, though there has been little formal investigation of such treatment of fallers.

The amount of balance and gait retraining required depends on the degree of instability and its causes, and the type of input will depend on whether the fallers confidence has been badly shaken by the fall. Some fallers seem unbothered by their balance problems, to the extent that they are overconfident and dangerous, lacking insight into their limitations. Many such will have a degree of cognitive impairment, or perceptual damage from strokes, and are often quite difficult to help (the 'I'll be all right when I get home' syndrome), though persistence and continued practice may eventually lead to some improvement. Balance retraining essentially follows the standard steps of concentrating first on sitting balance (static then dynamic), then moving onto standing balance (again static then dynamic). For each step, the difficulty of the balance task is gradually increased as the subject progresses and gains confidence. Some old people develop difficulty with standing upright following a period of illness, particularly if they have spent time in bed, and develop a marked backward lean, as if they have forgotten which way is up. This may be helped by plenty of 'standing practice' in a standing frame or standing against a hospital bed in its highest position, leaning forward slightly against pillows (Fig. 7.3). Providing them with a wheeled walking frame rather than a standard frame also helps to normalise stance and walking position.

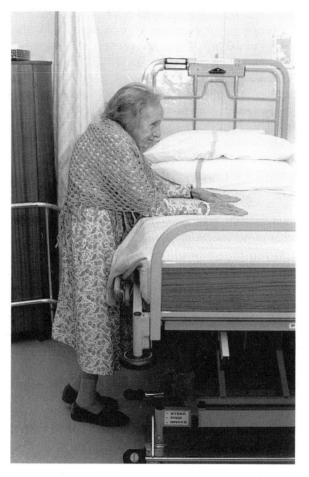

Fig. 7.3 'Backward-leaner' having her posture corrected by leaning forward against a hospital bed

Once balance and gait have improved, teaching someone how to get up after a fall is often useful. It is impossible to guarantee that further falls will not occur, but the ability to get up independently may avoid the potentially dangerous 'long lie' (Wild et al., 1981), and is often of psychological benefit to fallers, as it allows them to regain some degree of control over their situation. This approach has been used in a teaching pack for elderly people, their carers, and professionals working with the elderly (Walsall Health Authority, 1991).

Techniques for getting up from the floor following a fall are relatively simple and can be taught to elderly people at risk of falls (Fig. 7.4). The first thing to stress is that the faller should not rush but should try to relax and take his/her time. The important movements to practice are turning over from lying on the back, and getting on to hands and knees from a prone position. Then the faller can crawl to a raised surface such as a chair or bed, and use the raised surface to pull him/herself up, first on to one knee, then to a standing position. If the faller is unable to turn over onto his/her front, an alternative is to shuffle on the bottom to a chair and use that to pull or push up. It is usually helpful for carers to be taught how to assist the faller to get up using these techniques as well, since many carers, themselves elderly, risk injury when trying to lift the faller bodily from the floor. It would be sensible to allow patients in rehabilitation areas to get themselves up from the floor in this way if they fall on the ward (after a brief check for injury and with assistance if necessary from staff), to reinforce the teaching of self-reliance, rather than being 'picked up' by staff.

As yet, advice about physiotherapy for fallers is empirical rather than based firmly on reliable experimental studies. This is clearly an area which would benefit from further investigation.

Where the fear induced by falling has become debilitating, intervention by a clinical psychologist may be helpful. The psychological impact of falls should not be underestimated, but behavioural retraining or anxiety management may allow elderly fallers to come to terms with their tendency to fall without limiting their activity to an unacceptable degree. Learning to get up from the floor independently can improve morale and reduce the feeling of helplessness that frequent falling can induce.

The environment and falls

The dependency of advancing age is only partly due to intrinsic disease or physiological decline. The psychological, social and physical environments also play their part. Because ageing is expected to be associated with increasing frailty, dependency and social incompetence, problems that arise (which may be due to treatable disease or reversible disability) are accepted as inevitable and immutable, and the common response is restriction of activity and contraction of social horizons. Inactivity leads to atrophy and deterioration becomes irreversible.

The way in which society allows for such problems depends on its view of the value of those suffering. To a large extent, the dependence of children is expected, accepted and provided for by society, because providing for children is seen as an investment in the future. The dependency of the old, however, has no positive aspect, and is seen to presage inevitable deterioration, resulting in 'cost' for society, with the worry that society may not be able to 'afford' to support the dependent elderly.

As the competence of individuals decreases, environmental factors become increasingly important in their independence. If your vision is poor, making your way around depends on clearer visual clues than if your vision is good. Because the dependence of the elderly will have at least some environmental

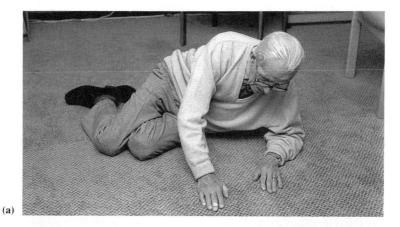

(a)

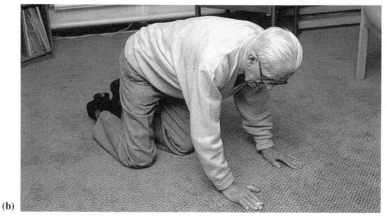

(b)

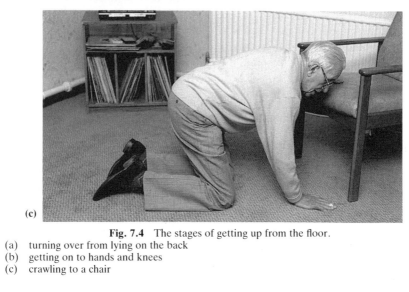

(c)

Fig. 7.4   The stages of getting up from the floor.
(a)   turning over from lying on the back
(b)   getting on to hands and knees
(c)   crawling to a chair

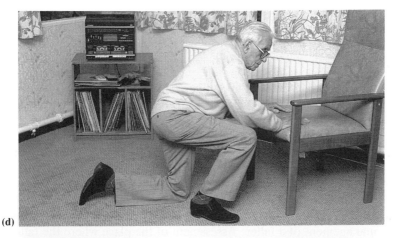

(d)

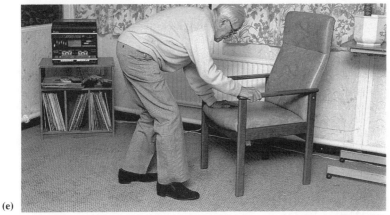

(e)

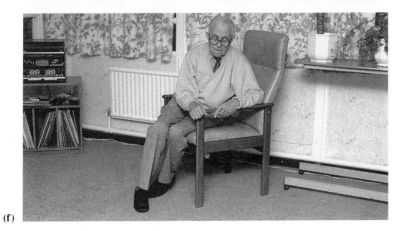

(f)

(d) using the chair to help get up onto one knee
(e) standing with the help of the chair
(f) sitting down to rest

aspects it is therefore necessary to identify and reduce the excess disability that is environmentally induced and does not reflect actual impairment, in order to maximise independence.

These principles are as true in the context of falls as they are in any aspect of the elderly and their health problems. Because falls are related to and affect mobility, environmental factors are particularly important, though in many cases they are only one (and often the least important) of many factors predisposing to falls. The role of the environment in causation of falls has already been discussed in Chapter 5, and the interaction between environmental factors and intrinsic factors (such as the age-related changes in gait making tripping over irregular paving stones more likely because the feet are not lifted sufficiently) is often more important than external factors alone in causing falls. It is therefore important to consider the role of the environment in the management of a faller. Assessment of the place where the faller lives and spends most of his/her time may provide diagnostic information, and may allow suggestions for the alteration of environmental factors which are adding to medical or functional problems.

However, the elderly person must retain control over changes to the environment, as a feeling of control over events is vital to maintaining psychological health. He/she must also be allowed to accept some risks. A completely risk-free environment is impossible, and we all choose to take risks every day of our lives, that choice being part of our control over our lives. Protecting elderly people against harm should not mean taking away their autonomy.

There are a number of specific areas in the home of an elderly faller which merit attention. A checklist such as that produced by the Centre for Policy on Ageing may be useful to highlight areas of risk and potential for improvement (Wynne-Harley, 1991).

Floors and floor coverings are obviously important as potential sources of tripping and slipping. The ideal floor for an elderly person with gait and mobility problems would have a non-slip surface, would not be polished and should have no irregularities. Carpets, particularly with underlay, may reduce risk of injury if a fall occurs but may be more difficult to negotiate, particularly if the pile is thick or a walking frame is used. However, a study comparing different sorts of floor covering found that elderly hospital inpatients walked faster on a carpeted than on a vinyl-tiled corridor (Willmott, 1986). The patterns and colours of floor coverings may also have an effect on mobility and safety, particularly on stairs (Archea, 1985). Those items of furniture which are used for stability when the elderly person is moving around the home need to be secure and stable, and obvious risks such as loose rugs and cluttered floor areas should be corrected if possible.

The movements involved in bending require a degree of flexibility, and may unbalance the body. They may therefore increase the risk of falling. For this reason, plugs and switches just above floor level may be difficult and potentially risky to reach. Thus, provision of raised plugs, and fires with

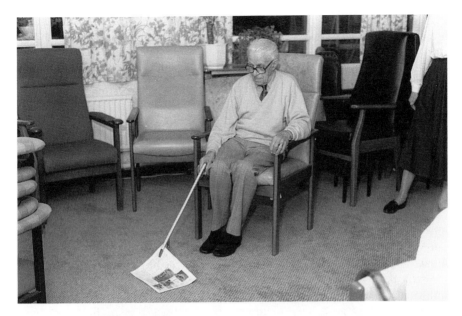

Fig. 7.5 A 'helping-hand' allows you to pick up objects from the floor without reaching or bending

controls on the top rather than the side may be safer and easier for the elderly person to manipulate. A 'helping hand' device can help someone reach objects on the floor without bending (Fig. 7.5). Lighting levels may need to be increased as the common visual problems of the elderly mean that higher light levels are needed to maintain effective vision (Cullinan et al., 1979). Glare, however, is poorly tolerated, so types of lighting may need to be altered to provide good, glare-free light, particularly at potentially dangerous (and often poorly lighted) sites such as stairs and corridors. In addition, light switches need to be easily accessible and clearly visible at points of entry to rooms. If someone regularly has to get up to the toilet at night it may be worth having a night light on continuously.

Bathrooms are often risky areas. Floors may be slippery, particularly if water is spilt on them. There may be loose mats on the floor, and the toilet may be too low to allow someone with a degree of muscle weakness to get up from sitting. As well as a raised toilet seat, provision of grab rails or a Scandia frame (Fig. 7.6) around the toilet may assist someone with poor mobility and balance to get on and off the toilet easily and safely. Separate toilets are often small, and entry and exit, particularly with a walking aid, may be difficult, as may manoeuvring to sit on the toilet. Altering hinges to allow doors to open outwards may make things easier.

Many old people find getting into and out of the bath difficult, and may stop using the bath because they fear falling whilst getting in or out. Provision of

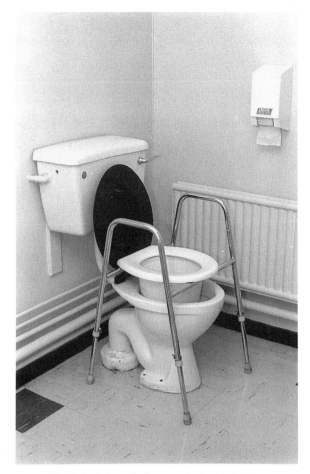

Fig. 7.6   A Scandia frame and raised toilet seat

grab rails around the bath, a non-slip mat in the bath and a bath seat may make such movements much safer.

Beds and chairs should be high enough and firm enough to allow safe transfers on and off. There may need to be a balance between a bed that is high enough to allow a frail elderly person to stand from sitting with ease, whilst being low enough to allow the legs to be lifted on to the bed without too much difficulty. Many living room chairs are low and soft, and may be difficult even for a fit young person to get out of. 'Ejector' chairs can sometimes help, particularly in those with arthritic hips and knees, but if balance is poor there is a risk that the person may be catapulted forward in an uncontrolled manner. Chairs with arms are safer and easier to get in and out of, so dining chairs without arms may cause problems.

Kitchens are again areas with many potential dangers. There is the risk of liquids being spilt on the floor, making the floor slippery; kitchen cupboards may be awkward to reach, requiring unbalanced movements; and cooking often requires movements whilst carrying heavy and/or hot utensils, when concentration on walking may be reduced. Many kitchens are poorly designed, even in purpose-built homes for the elderly. Simple interventions, such as placing commonly used utensils in cupboards which can easily be reached, and providing a trolley for putting things on to move them around the kitchen may improve safe mobility. A perching stool, to remove the need for standing whilst working in the kitchen, may also help.

Stairs are potentially dangerous areas. Walking up and down stairs requires a greater degree of effort than walking on the flat, and there is a risk of severe injury if a fall occurs. Handrails should ideally be on both sides of the stairs, and should be appropriately shaped for easy grasping. For those with poor vision, knobs at the ends of the rail will remind the subject that the top or bottom step is approaching. Providing two walking aids, one for upstairs and one for downstairs removes the need to carry a stick or frame up and down stairs.

If the faller lives alone there may need to be some consideration of provision of an alarm, to summon help if further falls occur. Warden controlled flats usually have a pull cord in each room, though in practice the pull cords are often tied up to keep them out of the way! A body-worn alarm is theoretically more effective, though again, elderly people do not always seem to be able to use them effectively if they fall. The main benefit of an alarm may be in reassuring carers and bolstering the confidence of the faller.

Footwear and clothing should be considered in the assessment. Poorly fitted or worn shoes or slippers may make tripping more likely, and providing appropriate footwear may improve mobility and safety. Similarly, trailing clothing can cause trips (Stall and Katz, 1987). Minor leg length discrepancy, perhaps because of arthritic hips or knees should be sought, and if present a shoe raise should be tried. However, if someone has got used to a minor inequality of leg lengths, correcting it may throw him/her off balance.

There is less that can be done about risky areas in the environment outside the home, particularly in public areas, which often seem to have been specifically designed to exacerbate the mobility problems of the elderly. Uneven and irregular paving stones and pathways are ubiquitous, pedestrian crossings do not allow sufficient time for those who walk slowly to cross safely, and moving hazards such as cyclists and skateboarders are not uncommon on pavements. Improvements in these areas require changes in public policy, but would enhance quality of life for the disabled of all ages.

Longer term management of a faller is essentially the secondary prevention of further falls and is considered in Chapter 9.

Fallers and the Accident and Emergency Department

This is an area where thorough assessment of elderly fallers is most important, since people presenting to the Accident Department will include those with significant illnesses, as well as those with serious injuries and more trivial falls. The degree of injury is not necessarily an indicator of the potential seriousness of the underlying medical problem. It is also an area where simple protocols can significantly improve management of many problems, including the elderly with falls.

Once the fallers condition has been stabilised, the casualty officer has to decide whether the patient is sufficiently ill or injured to require admission to hospital, which then requires a decision as to which speciality is best able to deal with the problem. Secondly, if the patient does not require admission, the casualty officer must decide what immediate management is appropriate, and whether action needs to be taken for longer term management of the problem. Important factors that need to be borne in mind include the tendency for falls to be one of the non-specific presentations of acute ill-health in the elderly, and the limited reserve of the elderly person to cope with the homoeostatic stresses of injury and illness.

Patients will fall into several groups: those who are significantly injured with or without acute illness; those who are not significantly injured but are acutely ill; those who are basically healthy and independent, with trivial or no significant injury and no acute illness; and those who are not significantly injured, not acutely ill, but frail and/or chronically ill. Those who are significantly injured are likely to need referral to orthopaedic or general surgeons, and those who are acutely ill to geriatricians or general physicians, and the basically healthy and non-injured can be discharged (though non-urgent referral for further assessment may be appropriate if they have had recurrent falls or the cause of their fall is not clear). The remaining group, usually very elderly and frail, can sometimes be difficult to manage appropriately. Ascertaining their social support circumstances, and carrying out a simple mobility assessment may allow discharge (again perhaps with outpatient referral) with reasonable confidence, but in some cases it is not possible to avoid admission to hospital for further assessment and observation, usually most appropriately carried out under the care of a geriatrician. 'Minor' fractures (e.g. Colle's fracture or fractured neck of humerus) are not generally thought to require inpatient treatment, but if they happen to a very frail old person, who when uninjured is only just able to look after him/herself, short-term admission to hospital may be required. Whether this should be under the care of orthopaedic surgeons or geriatricians is a question that often leads to a degree of conflict between the specialities, and should ideally be agreed by local negotiations.

In all circumstances, it is important to actually think about the cause of the

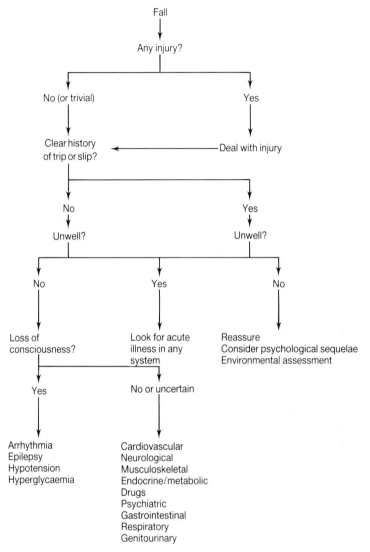

Fig. 7.7   Flowchart to aid the assessment and management of falls

fall, as this may make it clear whether the patient can be discharged or not. An algorithm such as that shown in Fig. 7.7 can aid assessment and management.

General practitioners and fallers

General (family) practitioners (GPs) are often the first port of call for elderly people who have fallen, and therefore assessment in a similar fashion to that carried out in Accident and Emergency Departments is often required. In addition, GPs are often those to whom worried carers of frequent fallers come. The general principles of assessment and management of fallers discussed above are clearly relevant, but there are specific areas of interest and influence which apply to GPs managing fallers.

The responsibility for referring elderly people with falls to appropriate hospital departments for further specialised assessment rests with GPs. They have an important role in educating the elderly and their carers about which problems are related to the ageing process and which may therefore be irreversible, and which problems may be amenable to medical or other treatment. A GP with a dismissive attitude to the health problems of the elderly, including falls ('it's just your age, dear') can have a major negative effect on quality of life and independence of the elderly in his/her care. Realistic assessment, either by the GP him/herself, or by referral to an appropriate specialist, of the factors underlying the tendency to fall and whether attention to these factors can reduce risk of further falls is the most important element of management of the faller.

General practitioners are also extremely important for the support of the frail elderly in their own homes, and helping to maintain independent existence of such patients may require a degree of selflessness on the part of the GP, as they often require more frequent and time-consuming care than their healthier peers. Continuing follow-up and regular reassessment of risk factors are important in maintaining optimum functioning and independence.

Elderly people often rely heavily on advice from their GP about whether it is sensible to remain at home or whether institutional care should be considered once they begin experiencing problems such as falls. Advising an elderly person to give up his or her home, and with it a substantial degree of autonomy, is a heavy responsibility and such a decision should not be taken lightly. Where the decision is appropriate GPs are often best placed to advise, since they often have extensive knowledge of the medical, social and psychological background to the problems. It is, however, probably true to say that the majority of requests for emergency or urgent placement in institutional care occur in situations where medical problems have arisen, and when appropriate management of the medical problems can be arranged, institutionalisation may be avoided. This is particularly true when the problem is a fall or repeated falls, since 'medical' factors are important causes.

Since the majority of drug prescribing occurs in the community by general practitioners, GPs have an important responsibility for rational prescribing. As discussed in Chapter 5, drugs are an important cause of falls, and avoidance as far as possible of drugs that increase risk of falling would do much to reduce overall rate of falling. In addition, drugs prescribed for the problems associated with falls, such as dizziness, may make things worse rather than better, and thoughtful assessment of elderly patients' symptoms may help avoid such difficulties.

References

Archea, J.C. (1985). Environmental factors associated with stair accidents by the elderly. *Clin Geriatr Med*. **1:** 555–568.

Burley, L.E. (1983). The joint geriatric orthopaedic service in south Edinburgh. In *Advanced Geriatric Medicine 3*. Caird, F.I. and Evans, J.G. (eds). London: Pitman.

Cullinan, T.R., Silver, J.H., Gould, E.S. and Irvine, D. (1979). Visual disability and home lighting. *Lancet*. **1:** 642–644.

Mathias, S., Nayak, U.S.L. and Isaacs, B. (1986). Balance in elderly patients: the 'get up and go' test. *Arch Phys Med Rehabil*. **67:** 387–389.

Obonyo, T., Drummond, M. and Isaacs, B. (1983). Domiciliary physiotherapy for old people who have fallen. *Int Rehabil Med*. **5:** 157–160.

Rubenstein, L.Z., Robbins, A.S., Schulman, B.L., Rosado, J., Osterweil, D. and Josephson, K.R. (1988). Falls and instability in the elderly. *J Am Geriatr Soc*. **36:** 266–278.

Stall, R. and Katz, P.R. (1987). Falls and ill-fitting clothing (letter). *J Am Geriatr Soc*. **35:** 959.

Tinetti, M.E. (1986). Performance-oriented assessment of mobility problems in elderly patients. *J Am Geriatr Soc*. **34:** 119–126.

Tinetti, M.E. and Ginter, S.F. (1988). Identifying mobility dysfunctions in elderly patients. Standard neuromuscular examination or direct assessment? *JAMA*. **259:** 1190–1193.

Walsall Health Authority (1991). *Falls – a positive approach*. Walsall, WHA.

Wild, D., Nayak, U.S.L. and Isaacs, B. (1981). How dangerous are falls in old people at home. *Br Med J*. **282:** 266–268.

Willmott, M. (1986). The effect of a vinyl floor surface and a carpeted floor surface upon walking in elderly hospital in-patients. *Age Ageing*. **15:** 119–120.

Wolf-Klein, G.P., Silverstone, F.A., Basavaraju, N., Foley, C.J., Pascaru, A. and Ma, P.-H. (1988). Prevention of falls in the elderly population. *Arch Phys Med Rehabil*. **69:** 689–691.

Wynne-Harley, D. (1991). *Living dangerously: risk-taking, safety and older people.*

Chapter 8 _____

Nursing aspects of falls and falling

Hospitalised and institutionalised elderly are at greater risk of falling than old people living in the community. Amongst these higher-risk groups the role of nurses in management of falls, identification of those prone to falling, and limitation of risk of falls is vital. This is reflected in the large nursing literature on the subject, which particularly covers the latter two of these three areas. The relationship between numbers or types of staff and frequency of falls has also been considered. The topic raises many questions about the responsibilities of nursing staff towards their elderly charges, and it becomes clear that nurses often view the situation differently from their medical colleagues. When a patient falls, nurses often feel that this reflects on their care of the patient, and this may result in much distress. This reaction is only partly due to the risk that they may be held legally responsible for injury to their patient, and more often reflects the personal and emotional involvement with the individual that frequently occurs as part of the close relationship between nurse and patient.

Staffing levels and falls

Findings from studies looking at the relationship between staff numbers and frequency of falls are sometimes conflicting. In some cases, a negative correlation between patient falls and number of staff has been found, with falls being commoner when staff levels are low (Fine, 1959). Others have argued that the availability of staff is the key factor (Morse et al., 1987), or that the competence, not the absolute number of staff, is important in reducing falls (Lynn, 1980). It has sometimes been noted that most falls occur when the largest number of staff are on duty (Sehested and Severin-Nielsen, 1977), which may partly be explained by a greater level of activity leading to more 'risky' activities. This is supported by an interesting study of the organisational and staff attitudinal determinants of falls in nursing home residents which found that the more involved the nursing staff were in their job, the more patient falls occurred. This was interpreted as being due to the fact that involved staff encouraged patients to be more active, so that more opportunities for falls arose. In addition, 'as staff attitudes toward the elderly became more positive, the frequency of falls increased'. '[S]taff with a more positive attitude were more inclined to encourage patients to be more independent, thus increasing the risk of falling' (Harris, 1989).

The role of nurses in the management of falls and fallers

Individual institutions have their own regulations and practices for the management of falls. If a fall has occurred, it is usually required that some form of incident or accident form is filled out, to document the circumstances of the fall and to indicate whether any injury has occurred. These documents are rarely of much help in the management of the fall or the faller, but their use means that frequency of falls in hospitals and other institutions caring for the elderly can be documented, which may be valuable as an audit measure. A more thoughtful collection of information at the time of a fall could, however, be useful to identify treatable causes of the fall and determine which fallers need medical attention, and might allow sensible risk reduction for many fallers.

There are several aspects of the accident form that need to be considered. Documenting the frequency of falls may be part of audit of quality of care of the institutionalised or hospitalised elderly (O'Brien et al., 1987); information may need to be collected for potential medico-legal requirements; and assessment of the faller is necessary to determine whether injury has occurred or medical intervention is required. For the majority of accident forms in use, the second of these elements predominates. There is often little inquiry about the cause of the fall, and guidance about which fallers might require medical attention, either because of injury, or because of the event(s) causing the fall, is rarely included. In hospitals there is often a requirement that medical staff be informed about the fall, and in British hospitals, significant amounts of junior medical staff time and effort in geriatric units is spent seeing (or at least being informed about) patients who have fallen, and signing accident forms. The utility of such effort is rarely questioned, but one suspects that the point of the activity is that assessment of a faller is seen to be done (for medico-legal reasons). The procedure rarely seems to be carried out to genuinely understand why the fall occurred or to reduce the risk of further falls.

Because falls are so common in the institutionalised elderly, and because only a small proportion result in significant injury, it would be sensible to use an accident (or perhaps more appropriately incident) form which attempted to identify those fallers who would benefit from further assessment, both by nursing and medical staff. This would help to determine what caused the fall, whether intervention was required to modify factors (both intrinsic and

---

INCIDENT FORM

A. General particulars
  Date and time of incident
  Patient name (and perhaps other details, e.g. age, sex, etc.)

B. Particulars of the incident
  Type of incident (fall, other accident)
  Was incident witnessed?
  If so, by whom?
  Description of incident (from patient and/or witnesses).
Particular factors to note:
  What was he/she doing at the time of the incident?
  Was this a normal activity for him/her either alone or with assistance? (i.e. *did incident happen whilst patient was doing something that he/she should normally be able to do without problems)
  *Any symptoms prior to incident (e.g. chest pain, 'dizziness', palpitations)?
  any obvious environmental factors (e.g. wet floor, loose carpet, faulty equipment etc)?

C. The patient
  *Any obvious injuries?
  *Any change from usual functional status (e.g. continence, dependence, mobility)?
  *Does he/she seem well?

D. Action taken

---

*These factors may suggest that assessment by medical staff would be helpful.

Fig. 8.1 Incident form

environmental) putting the patient at risk of falls, and whether there was significant injury requiring treatment. It is also important to use a form which is simple and quick to fill in so that it does not impose unnecessary extra work on hard-pressed nursing and care staff. The sort of form suggested by some workers in the field is very full and inclusive (Barbieri, 1983), but would take some time to fill in, and would be unlikely to be used other than in research situations. A form such as that in Fig. 8.1 might be more effective than many currently in use.

Identification of those prone to falls

There have been a number of studies to try to identify the 'fall-prone' patient, or to identify particular factors such as staffing levels or time of day which are associated with a high risk of falls. A number of common themes arise. Hospital inpatients are more prone to fall in the early stages of their hospitalisation, presumably because of unfamiliarity with their new surroundings, and falls tend to occur at times of greatest activity on the ward. As discussed above, there is some relationship between levels of staffing and frequency of falls, though if staffing levels are very low falls may be less common, probably because activity is discouraged (Morris and Isaacs, 1980). Numerous medical factors have been identified as indicating a high risk of falling amongst the elderly in hospital (and in fact amongst younger patients as well). The commonest are neurological and cardiovascular problems, impairment of cognitive function, problems with gait, and multiple diagnoses. Most studies are retrospective in nature, and the populations studied are variable and usually not clearly described. Generalisation of their results is therefore not always easy. On the basis of good epidemiological information about factors increasing risk of falls it is possible to produce a 'fall risk score' for various types of hospitalised or institutionalised elderly, though at present there is little information from prospective studies that such scores are effective tools for preventing falls. Once again, long complicated forms which some have advocated (Fife et al., 1984) are unlikely to be used consistently outside research units.

A simple fall risk score (Fig. 8.2) for continuing care patients showed some

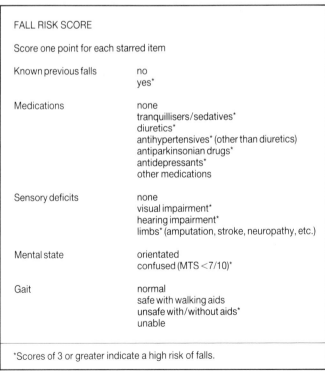

Fig. 8.2 Fall risk score

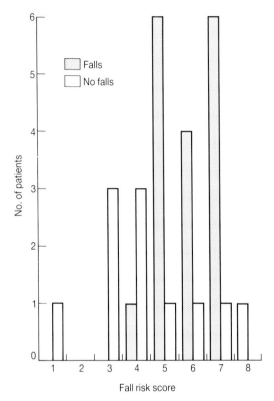

Fig. 8.3 Relationship between fall risk score and presence of falls in the previous year amongst 28 patients in an NHS continuing care ward

degree of association with number of falls in the previous year (Fig. 8.3), and is currently being tested for its use to predict likelihood of falling (Downton, 1992).

The hospital environment and falls

Considering that most old people in hospital are physically and/or mentally frail, and that the hospital environment is supposed to be 'safe' and protecting them against harm, many objects with which they come into contact during their stay in hospital are poorly designed, and seem, in fact, to be devised to increase risk of falls and injuries. Beds, chairs and lockers which move when they are used for support, 'geriatric chairs' which are unstable when the occupant steps on the footplate and which have numerous protruding elements to bang against (Fig. 8.4), and wheelchairs with footrests which are ideal to trip over when raised are widespread, not to mention the various hazards produced by objects left on the floor (either deliberately or by

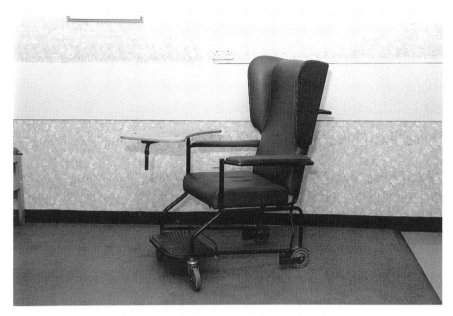

Fig. 8.4   A potentially dangerous 'geriatric chair'

mistake), such as urine bottles, cleaning buckets and warning cones on wet floors. Tip-back chairs, which thankfully are much less common now on hospital wards than they used to be, are very likely to lead to balance problems and a backward-leaning stance, increasing risk of falling. In addition, they are likely to lead to sensory deprivation and disorientation because of long periods spent staring at a blank ceiling.

The various activities and equipment associated with elimination seem to be particularly risky. Trailing catheter bags, particularly if full will very effectively inhibit normal walking. Incontinence of urine onto a shiny vinyl hospital floor produces an extremely slippery surface. The urgency of micturition experienced by many older people results in a situation where care is unlikely to be taken in getting to the toilet. Dribbling incontinence of urine and urgency of micturition are a potentially lethal combination as the old man with prostate trouble tries to get to the toilet across the wet and slippery floor!

One study of falls and accidents in hospital found that about a quarter of incidents occurred in association with toileting. 'The large number of accidents involving toileting may reflect the amount of time spent in such activity but also emphasises the hazards of "transferring" (an unfamiliar manoeuvre for most people) on to a commode (an unfamiliar apparatus for most people) or of making the long walk through unfamiliar surroundings to an unfamiliar lavatory and back as well as organising the act of toileting itself' (Watkins and Robson, 1981).

Inappropriate footwear and trailing clothing are other potential causes of falls. In hospitals where patients wear hospital clothing rather than their own (or where frequent incontinence or soiling means that their own clothing is not sufficient) items may not fit adequately and there may be a lack of belts or braces to hold up trousers. If your balance or walking skills have not yet returned to normal, the gentle descent of your trousers as you walk across the ward is very likely to result in tripping or falling.

Limiting the risk of (further) falls

Because it is widely recognised that the elderly, particularly the frail elderly in hospital or institutional care, are at risk of falls and other accidents, one of the aims of the institution is to limit these risks as far as possible. Nursing staff in particular are given responsibility for this aspect of care. This is not a straightforward responsiblity and there are conflicting demands on nursing staff. Sometimes the interests of patients and their relatives or carers diverge and anyone who deals with elderly fallers will be familiar with the sometimes unrealistic demands from relatives that there should be no risk of further falls. There is also conflict between the 'medical' and 'civil liberties' models (Schafer, 1985). The medical model is to take action as soon as possible and to minimise the possibility of harmful effects. The civil liberties model is that procedural safeguards are required if there is a proposal to deprive someone of freedom, with the onus of proof resting with those who would restrict liberty. The medical model may be based on compassion and a desire to help; however it is paternalistic, potentially controlling and demeaning. If a person is labelled as not capable of rational choice, this often means that he/she is viewed as no longer fully a person.

In both acute and chronic care areas, there is a paradox that staff are expected to have an enabling function in relation to the independence of their patients, but are simultaneously expected to protect patients against risks of various kinds. This is particularly so in rehabilitation areas, where staff encourage patients to increase their activities, and to carry out these activities with decreasing levels of supervision. The patients may be initially unsafe, and therefore at very high risk of falling, but protecting them from falls would undermine and inhibit the rehabilitation. This balance between reduction of risk of falling and maintenance of independence is an issue of paramount importance and is dealt with in different ways in North America and the United Kingdom.

In the United States and Canada there has always been much wider use of 'restraint' of patients (of all ages) to limit risk of injury from falls and accidents, to the extent that 7–10 per cent of general hospital patients are restrained at any one time (Frengley and Mion, 1986), whereas in the United Kingdom, such restraint, although used to some extent, is not so common. A demonstration of the difference between the two parts of the world is that types of equipment available and commonly used in the USA, such as vest restraints, are unknown in the UK. There are, however, disturbing sugges- tions recently that physical and pharmacological restraint of residents in private residential and nursing homes in the UK is becoming increasingly common. In view of the growing tendency in the UK for continuing care for frail elderly people to be provided outside hospital, and largely in the private sector, these suggestions are worrying.

Current knowledge about falls in the elderly indicates that intrinsic factors are important (perhaps the most important) causes of falls. From this it follows that if one is trying to minimise falls, and attempts to identify reversible intrinsic causes of falls are unsuccessful, then preventing falls means preventing the activities during which falls occur. If you cannot reduce the liability to fall, then you must reduce the opportunity. This approach has been followed particularly in hospitals and institutions where elderly are cared for on a long-term basis.

Falls tend to occur on movement, and particular movements are seen as especially risky. Movements that involve change in position, such as getting out of bed or getting up from a chair, are viewed as potentially dangerous. It is felt by some that if patients can be persuaded to stay in a chair during the day and in bed at night, and not get up and walk without supervision then most falls can be avoided. There is some evidence in favour of this view. When a falls prevention programme made use of a device which alerted nursing staff whenever a patient got out of bed or up from a chair, the incidence of falls fell by 60 per cent over two years (Morton, 1989).

The problem with this sort of approach is that monitoring and supervising activity to this extent necessarily limits autonomy and results in patients remaining relatively immobile, which is recognised to have its own complica- tions, and may paradoxically increase risk of falling (Miller, 1975). Because of concerns about medico-legal responsibilities, nursing staff may feel compelled to rely on excessive levels of supervision and restriction of patients felt to be at risk. 'Once alerted [to high risk of falling] our nurses look in on the at-risk patient every time they pass his room. They pad his bed's side rail if appropriate, and keep all the rails up . . . Whenever the patient is out of bed, they keep him within view or in a Geri chair or Posey vest' (Morton, 1989).

Use of restraint devices to reduce or prevent falls

'Every year in North America thousands, perhaps tens of thousands, of elderly patients are subjected to involuntary restrictions on their liberty. The restrictions may be physical (e.g. locked rooms, jackets, wristlets or bands) or pharmacologic (e.g. psychotropic drugs)' (Schafer, 1985). Preventing falls is cited as one of the main reasons for restraining patients, being mentioned in up to 90 per cent of cases (Strumpf and Evans, 1988). There is a big difference in the frequency with which physical restraint is used in North America and

Europe, and it is likely that different medico-legal environments contribute to this contrast (Cushing, 1989). There is little information about the frequency with which pharmacological restraint is used on either side of the Atlantic.

Several issues are raised when the use of restraint to reduce the risk of falling is considered. What evidence is there that restraint prevents falls or reduces risk of falling? What are the effects of restraints on the general well-being of patients? How does the use of restraints affect nursing (and other staff) attitudes in general and in particular towards their patients? The rationale for use of restraints includes reducing the risk of injury, controlling patients exhibiting confusion, maintaining integrity of treatment plans for confused and agitated patients, providing physical security, and limiting movement. However, protective devices may precipitate or exacerbate many problems, including falls, for which they are applied. Restraint seldom eliminates risk of injury, and patients are often very adept at freeing themselves from restraints. Restraints may themselves cause risk to the patient, and have resulted in fatal injury (Dube and Mitchell, 1986).

Cot-sides (bed-rails) are commonly used for elderly patients felt to be at risk of falling, particularly in North America, where they are almost routine for patients aged more than 65 or 70. The absence of cot-sides may be taken by American judges and juries as evidence of negligence. There is, however, no evidence that cot-sides prevent falls, whilst there is good evidence that they do not (Lynn, 1980; Rubenstein et al., 1983). 'When used with a confused or restless patient, cotsides probably do not diminish his risk of falling, may increase his confusion and distress, and certainly ensure, whether he is confused or lucid, that if he does fall it will be from a greater height' (Anonymous, 1984). In a study of accidents in a geriatric department in the UK, cot-sides were involved in 10 per cent of incidents. 'One patient climbed over the top, the others crawled to the end of the bed and fell head-first to the floor. There was no accident recorded during the night involving a patient trying to get out of bed by herself with no cotsides in place' (Tinker, 1979). It is interesting that in Britain, where cot-sides are more selectively used, hospital fall-fracture rates are lower than in the United States (Rubenstein et al., 1983).

Although (or perhaps because) restraints are frequently used on patients with cognitive impairment (either acute or chronic), patients often have a profound response to being restrained. A lack of insight consequent on the cognitive impairment may mean that their understanding of the reason for restraint is reduced or absent, and this may increase distress. Restraints may intensify disorganised behaviour, and contribute to sensory deprivation, loss of self-image and increased dependency. They may increase confusion by limiting communication, increase disorientation, and precipitate regressive behaviour or withdrawal. The restrained patient tends to be viewed by others as disturbed, dangerous or mentally incompetent.

A study of the responses of restrained patients to their experiences found a wide range of reactions, most of them negative. They included anger, fear, humiliation, demoralisation, and discomfort. Some patients reacted with resistance or denial, and a few agreed that restraint had been necessary. Patients remembered the experience of restraint for a long time after discharge (Strumpf and Evans, 1988).

Nursing staff are often ambivalent about restraining patients at risk of falls or other harm. They are under some pressure to ensure the safety of their patients, sometimes to the exclusion of all other considerations, whilst being aware of the absurdity of achieving safety at the expense of the very goals being pursued. '[He] will lose his mobility if he breaks a hip, so we will tie him down to prevent the loss of mobility' (Silver, 1987). They are also under pressure for medico-legal reasons, being not uncommonly held responsible for broken hips, particularly in North America. However, the use of restraint often leads to distress amongst those required to apply it. A study of nurse responses to using restraint identified many different reactions, but the majority were negative (anxiety, guilt, frustration, inadequacy, etc.) or neutral (surprise, absurdity, resignation), and very few were positive (DiFabio, 1981). Nurses recognise behavioural effects (attempts to remove restraints, agitation, resistance) and emotional effects (unhappiness, anger) on their patients when physical restraint is used, but may feel powerless to do otherwise. Patients who had been restrained came up with more alternatives to restraint than their nurses when asked about their experiences (Strumpf and Evans, 1988).

It is clear that use of physical restraint (and pharmacological restraint, though there is much less information about this) is ineffective in preventing falls, and has negative effects on patients and nurses. The reason for its continued use, particularly in North America, has more to do with legal constraints than medical indications, and use of restraint to prevent falls is inappropriate, damaging, and indicative of an overprotective and infantilising attitude to the elderly. '[F]alls could most effectively be prevented if all patients were given maximum doses of phenothiazines and cotsides were regularly fortified with the pig-nets formerly lashed over the tops of beds of restless elderly patients. The objectives of care for the elderly must include the fostering of rehabilitation and independence and these objectives are incompatible with the total prevention of falls' (Anonymous, 1984).

A more enlightened approach to preventing falls in hospitalised and institutionalised elderly

This could include a number of elements. It would be sensible to screen all those at risk for treatable causes of falls, at the time of their admission to a unit, and perhaps on a regular basis thereafter. A simple fall-risk score could be used in the way that the Norton score is used to identify those at risk of developing pressure sores. Each patient's level of risk for falls would thus be individually assessed and a programme to ameliorate risk factors devised. The unit should aim to promote independence in all patients as far as possible, and it is extremely important to educate relatives and carers about the aims of the unit, particularly where the objective is to rehabilitate the patient for discharge home. Staff, patients and relatives should be made aware that it is impossible to remove all risk of falling – a rehabilitation unit which does not have some falls is not rehabilitating its patients. This point should probably be stressed in ward policies, as relatives often have unrealistic expectations about the safety of hospitals.

In situations where a rehabilitation unit is particularly concerned with dealing with those who have had falls (for example an orthopaedic rehabilitation unit) consideration should be given to using falls experienced by patients during their rehabilitation on the unit as opportunities to practice getting up independently. If the faller can try to get up on his/her own after a fall, in a relatively safe and supervised situation, this may help him/her to face a return home with more confidence.

Falls as an audit measure

It has been suggested that frequency of falls in long term care institutions is a useful measure for auditing quality of care. As discussed above, there does seem to be a relationship between staff numbers, skill mix and fall frequency, but understaffing may paradoxically reduce falls because fewer activities are undertaken. A major difficulty is that because falls are very clearly multifactorial, with an enormously wide variety of potential precipitants and predisposing factors, drawing conclusions from figures obtained from small groups of patients (such as the occupants of a single or a few long-term care units) is difficult and potentially misleading. Another problem is that for any individual patient, risk of falling may vary quite considerably from day to day, because of the effect of 'short-term' risk factors and alterations in environmental risk. However, overall trends, particularly if obtained from larger groups of patients, may have some use as measures of quality of care.

It must be stressed again that it is impossible to prevent all falls and accidents, and that attempts to minimise falls can result in restriction of activity and autonomy to an unacceptable degree. Therefore, although a unit with a high rate of falls and accidents may be one in which risk factors are not being adequately assessed and rectified, an unusually low accident rate might suggest a unit where activities of patients are too restricted.

References

Anonymous (1984). Cotsides – protecting whom against what? (Editorial). *Lancet.* **2:** 383–384.
Barbieri, E.B. (1983). Patient falls are not patient accidents. *J Gerontol Nurs.* **9:** 165–173.

Cushing, M. (1989). Finding fault when patients fall. *Am J Nurs*. **89**: 808–809.

DiFabio, S. (1981). Nurse's reactions to restraining patients. *Am J Nurs*. **81**: 973–975.

Downton, J.H. (1992). Predicting falls in continuing care patients. (Manuscript in preparation.)

Dube, A. and Mitchell, E. (1986). Accidental strangulation from vest restraints. *JAMA*. **256**: 2725–2726.

Fife, D.D., Solomon, P. and Stanton, M. (1984). A risk/falls program: code orange for success. *Nurs Management*. **15**: 50–53.

Fine, W. (1959). An analysis of 277 falls in hospital. *Gerontol Clin*. **1**: 292–300.

Frengley, J.D. and Mion, L.C. (1986). Incidence of physical restraints on acute general medical wards. *J Am Geriatr Soc*. **34**: 565–568.

Harris, P.B. (1989). Organizational and staff attitudinal determinants of falls in Nursing Home residents. *Med Care*. **27**: 737–749.

Lynn, F.H. (1980). Incidents: need they be accidents? *Am J Nurs*. **80**: 1098–1101.

Miller, M.B. (1975). Iatrogenic and nurisgenic effects of prolonged immobilization of the ill aged. *J Am Geriatr Soc*. **23**: 360–369.

Morris, E.V. and Isaacs, B. (1980). The prevention of falls in a geriatric hospital. *Age Ageing*. **9**: 181–185.

Morse, J.M., Tylko, S.J. and Dixon, H.A. (1987). Characteristics of the fall-prone patient. *Gerontologist*. **27**: 516–522.

Morton, D. (1989). Five years of fewer falls. *Am J Nurs*. **89**: 204–205.

O'Brien, B.L., O'Such, D.J. and Palette, S.V. (1987). Setting realistic goals for quality assurance monitoring: patient falls versus patient days. *QRB*. **13**: 339–342.

Rubenstein, H.S., Miller, F.H., Postels, S. and Evans, H.B. (1983). Standards of medical care based on consensus rather than evidence: the case of routine bedrail use for the elderly. *Law Med Health Care*. **11**: 271–276.

Schafer, A. (1985). Restraints and the elderly: when safety and autonomy conflict. *Can Med Assoc J*. **132**: 1257–1260.

Sehested, P. and Severin-Nielsen, T. (1977). Falls by hospitalised elderly patients: causes, prevention. *Geriatrics*. **32**: 101–108.

Silver, M. (1987). Using restraint. *Am J Nurs*. **87**: 1414–1415.

Strumpf, N.E. and Evans, L.K. (1988). Physical restraint of the hospitalized elderly: perceptions of patients and nurses. *Nurs Res*. **37**: 132–137.

Tinker, G.M. (1979). Accidents in a geriatric department. *Age Ageing*. **8**: 196–198.

Watkins, J.S. and Robson, P. (1981). The hazards of rehabilitation. *Ann Roy Coll Surg Engl*. **63**: 386–389.

Chapter 9 _____

Prevention of falls

With a problem of the magnitude of falls amongst elderly people, with the functional and economic consequences that have been demonstrated, thought needs to be given to whether either falls or their consequences can be prevented. Prevention is made more difficult by the multiplicity of causes of falls, and the interaction of intrinsic and environmental factors, but a completely nihilistic attitude cannot be justified. A number of small-scale studies have demonstrated that thorough assessment of elderly fallers, and correction of alterable factors predisposing to falls can reduce frequency of further falls (Wolf-Klein et al., 1988; Morton, 1989).

The question of primary prevention is more difficult, however. It has been estimated that even in elderly people at high risk of further falls, large numbers of people would have to be 'treated' to prevent one hip fracture (Isaacs, 1985). This makes rigorous assessment of prevention programmes using clear endpoints such as fractures difficult because of the large numbers of subjects required to demonstrate benefit.

Primary prevention

Although primary prevention of falls and their complications is a mammoth task, and may not in practice be cost-effective, consideration of various aspects of primary prevention is useful to provide pointers to areas which could provide benefit for elderly fallers and potential fallers.

Identifying those at risk

Several 'fall risk scores' have been devised to try to identify those at particularly high risk of falling who might benefit from preventive action. The best known of these is based on institutionalised elderly, and includes mobility score, distant vision, hearing, morale score, mental status score, back extension, orthostatic blood pressure, medications and activities of daily living score (Tinetti et al., 1986). Unfortunately the elderly in institutional care are not typical of the elderly generally, and the score may therefore be of limited relevance for community-living old people. The sorts of people who require long term care are those with high dependency and multiple deficits, and in terms of the factors that have been identified retrospectively, they would almost all be classed as being at high risk of falling (Fife et al., 1984). In 'free-range' elderly, sensitivity and specificity of such scores is too low for them to be of very much practical use (Downton and Andrews, 1991). There is certainly a strong argument, however, for assessing elderly people entering institutional care for factors increasing risk of initial or recurrent falls. The value of regular monitoring is demonstrated by a study of institutionalised subjects with Alzheimer's disease in whom a changing level of dependency was a clear risk factor for falls (Brody et al., 1984).

Identifying environmental risks

Almost all falls have an environmental element and there may be some benefit in assessing the environment, either of an individual elderly person, or generally, to identify obvious risk factors for falls. The public environment is in the main not very 'elderly friendly', and measures to improve potential danger spots, such as uneven paving stones, pavement surfaces which are slippery when wet, or areas with poor lighting could reduce risk of falling and improve quality of life for elderly people by increasing their confidence to venture outside.

There is unfortunately a difference between identifying environmental risks and doing something about them. On an individual level, many elderly people are resistant to making changes in their surroundings which would reduce their risk of falling or injury, particularly if it means altering a longstanding lifestyle or place of residence. As far as the public environment is concerned, changes to make areas more accessible and safer for the elderly (which would also help younger disabled people as well) have financial implications which local and national governments are not always willing to countenance.

Screening for potential risk factors

In the United Kingdom, general practitioners now have an obligation to offer screening once a year to all people aged 75 and over. There has been much debate about the utility and cost-effectiveness of this screening programme, but it could be used to look for potential risk factors for falls. A simple assessment of vision, gait and mobility and appropriateness of regular medication could identify some, and perhaps many, of those at high risk of falls, and intervention in these areas could reduce risk of falling. A good standard of primary care for all elderly people to limit the amount of unnecessary medication, and to identify and deal appropriately with treatable 'age-related' illnesses such as Parkinson's disease, cataract, arthritis and congestive heart failure could potentially avoid (or at least defer) a proportion of falls.

Population approach to primary prevention

There is some evidence that population measures to improve general level of fitness may reduce risk of falling, though possibly at the risk of increased injury in those who do fall (Speechley and Tinetti, 1991), although others have argued that increased exercise could substantially reduce risk of hip fracture (Law et al., 1991). There is evidence that exercise programmes increase bone density in young and elderly subjects, and that elderly people who exercise regularly have higher bone density than their sedentary peers. In addition, regular exercise may maintain neuromuscular function and protective reflexes and possibly also cognitive function (Molloy et al., 1988). Lower limb weakness (particularly ankle dorsiflexion) is an important risk factor for falls and fractures (Aniansson et al., 1984; Whipple et al., 1987), and this could potentially be improved by regular exercise.

It is clear that strategies to reduce osteoporosis could reduce fracture rates, and this approach is being followed by many physicians in Europe and North America, via hormone replacement therapy for post-menopausal women. There is no doubt that treating post-menopausal women with oestrogens reduces the bone loss that occurs after the menopause, and maintains bone mass for as long as oestrogen is continued. It has been argued that temporary hormone replacement treatment after the menopause will have a lasting beneficial effect on bone mass (Christiansen et al., 1981). However, once hormone replacement therapy is stopped, accelerated bone loss occurs in the same way as after natural menopause (Fig. 9.1), or possibly at a faster rate (Lindsay et al., 1978), and within a few years the degree of bone loss has reached that likely to produce a high risk of fracture in an unprotected fall. In order to prevent hip fractures hormone replacement therapy would have to be continued indefinitely, or at least for longer than is presently common.

There is now fairly strong evidence that increasing calcium intake reduces age-related bone loss, and may in fact prevent bone loss altogether (Heaney, 1990). However, if high calcium intake is not maintained, the benefit is lost. The levels of calcium intake required to prevent bone loss are substantially higher than could be obtained by simple dietary adjustment, and would require pharmacological supplementation. If it is proposed to prevent fractures by treatment of all elderly women, and possibly elderly men in addition, with calcium supplements, the financial implications are substantial.

Secondary prevention

Many of the preventive strategies discussed above are also appropriate in the prevention of further falls in those who have already fallen. Because those who have already had at least one fall have a risk of falling double that of non-fallers, it may be more cost-effective to concentrate preventive measures on this group. In addition, having had a fall may make someone more amenable to making environmental changes to reduce risk.

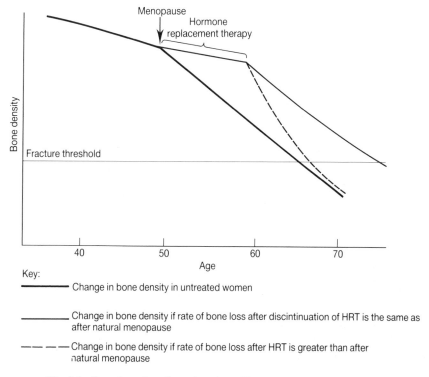

Key:

———— Change in bone density in untreated women

———— Change in bone density if rate of bone loss after discintinuation of HRT is the same as after natural menopause

— — — Change in bone density if rate of bone loss after HRT is greater than after natural menopause

Fig. 9.1 Bone loss after discontinuation of hormone replacement therapy

Identifying causes of previous falls and correcting them if possible

This is the most important aspect of secondary prevention, but failure to do this occurs with depressing regularity. Few old people presenting to Accident and Emergency Departments following a fall have any consistent inquiry into why they fell, and the ageist attitude that falls are to be expected in the elderly adds to the problem. Even geriatricians may dismiss falls as unavoidable. There is always a reason why someone falls, and a brief but thoughtful assessment will identify many of the treatable factors that have contributed to the fall. It is usually possible to identify in such patients one or more factors which increase their risk of falling, and modification of such factors can reduce risk of further falls.

Environmental risks

Assessment of the fallers abilities at home by an occupational therapist and a physiotherapist may be useful to identify obvious risk factors, though the faller may not be prepared to do anything about them. The question of acceptable risk and maintaining autonomy is discussed further below.

If falls are unavoidable, consider ways of preventing or limiting injury

In some elderly people there will remain a substantial risk of further falls despite the best efforts of medical, nursing and paramedical staff. Consideration should thus be given to limiting risk of injury. Any suggestions will have to be individually tailored to the situation of the faller, but factors worth considering might include carpeting high risk areas such as kitchens and bathrooms, providing chairs in strategic areas if falls occur with a preceding 'warning', thus allowing the faller to sit down rather than fall down, and so on. As a very last resort it may be necessary to restrict activity. Teaching the faller to get up from the floor may help by reducing the risk of a 'long lie' and by allowing the faller to retain an element of control, thus mitigating some of the confidence-sapping effects of falling.

Providing alarms

In those at high risk of continuing falls, particularly if they are not able to get up from the floor independently, provision of an alarm, preferably a body-worn one, can allow help to be summoned if a fall occurs. This is often a great comfort to fallers and their relatives and carers. Various types of alarms are now available, sometimes linked to 'mobile wardens', sometimes working via the telephone network.

Case report

A 91 year-old retired university lecturer was referred for assessment following a fall because of family concern about deterioration of balance. He had been riding a bicycle until the year before, but a few months previously had slipped on leaves in the garden, and had become aware of feeling less stable on his feet. He used two sticks outside, but largely used furniture to balance inside the house. His house was rather cluttered with furniture, and there were trailing wires and loose rugs on the floor. He had had a hip replacement 15 years previously, and now had evidence of moderate osteoarthritis of the other hip apparent on X-ray, though symptoms of pain and restriction of movement were mild. Further assessment revealed a mild degree of confusion, and loss of vibration sensation below the iliac crests, but no other neurological impairment, and examination was otherwise normal. His balance problems were probably due to reduction of proprioceptive input because of age-related peripheral nerve impairment and joint damage, and he was reassured that his arthritic hip did not need operative treatment at present.

He had an extensive network of friends and neighbours who visited regularly, and though he no longer cooked for himself he had a hot meal at a luncheon club five days a week. His daughter was expressing concern about the risk of further falls at home, and wondering about whether he should go into a residential home. It was explained that the mental and physical stimulation he received by staying at home were likely to keep him fitter than formal physiotherapy, and that relocation would be likely to provoke mental and physical deterioration. He was provided with a pendant alarm, and an attempt was made to make his home environment a little safer by removing some of the items he was at risk of tripping over. Although it was not possible to reduce his intrinsic risk of falling the assessment allowed him to be supported in his wish to remain at home, and reassured his daughter that it was reasonable to allow him to do so.

For both primary and secondary prevention it would be helpful to develop appropriate assessment schedules both for the person at risk of falls and for their environment. For these to be useful (and actually used!) they must be simple and quick to fill in, relevant, and regularly monitored and audited. What must be avoided, however, is taking risk reduction to extremes so that the autonomy of the faller is compromised. Unhelpful comments such as 'it is clear that patients with an impaired gait must be given walking aids or a wheelchair and not permitted to ambulate in this manner' (Morse et al., 1987) are common, and the attitudes which underlie such comments are widespread. An extensive discussion of the issues of risk and autonomy can be found in a report produced by the Centre for Policy on Ageing, and the following points are from that report, summarising the question of risk and 'at risk'.

The unthinking acceptance of age stereotypes is a threat to the independence of many older people. Families and the 'caring' professions must appreciate the difference between an individual's risky action or lifestyle which are chosen, and the state of being genuinely at risk.

Maintenance of the autonomy of the individual should be paramount. Anxiety in the minds of others should be regarded as a secondary consideration normally capable of resolution. When an older person appears to be at risk, the specific dangers and problems should be identified, their implications discussed with the individual and, wherever possible, reduced to an acceptable level without major changes in lifestyle.

Health and welfare professionals should adopt a positive attitude to risk-taking by older people in all settings. Their role should be to assist in informing public opinion of the normality of independence in older age and to encourage intergenerational acceptance, [and] to ensure people in the Third Age (post-work, active independence) have access to practical advice and information upon which to base their own decisions about lifestyle, risk-taking and safety' (Wynne-Harley, 1991).

Although the above comments are largely concerned with elderly people living at home, it is important to carry over such attitudes into the care of elderly in institutional settings. A paternalistic view is often taken that such people are no longer able to make sensible decisions about 'lifestyle, risk-taking and safety', and their autonomy is often severely restricted. Maintaining an acceptable quality of life for institutionalised elderly means accepting that it is not possible to remove all risks of falling, and allowing 'risky' behaviour when doing so means that quality of life is increased.

References

Aniansson, A., Zetterberg, C., Hedberg, M. and Henriksson, K.G. (1984). Impaired muscle function with aging. A background factor in the incidence of fractures of the proximal end of the femur. *Clin Orth Rel Res*. **191**: 193–201.

Brody, E.M., Kleban, M.H., Moss, M.S. and Kleban, F. (1984). Predictors of falls among institutionalised women with Alzheimers disease. *J Am Geriatr Soc*. **32**: 877–882.

Christiansen, C., Christiansen, M.S. and Transbol, I. (1981). Bone mass in postmenopausal women after withdrawl of oestrogen/gestagen replacement therapy. *Lancet*. **1**: 459–461.

Downton, J.H. and Andrews, K. (1991). Prevalence, characteristics and factors associated with falls among the elderly living at home. *Aging*. **3**: 219–228.

Fife, D.D., Solomon, P. and Stanton, M. (1984). A risk/falls program: code orange for success. *Nurs Management*. **15**: 50–53.

Heaney, R.P. (1990). Osteoporosis made easy (Editorial). *J Am Geriatr Soc*. **38**: 1159–1160.

Isaacs, B. (1985). Clinical and laboratory studies of falls in old people. Prospects for prevention. *Clin Geriatr Med*. **1**: 513–520.

Law, M.R., Wald, N.J. and Meade, T.W. (1991). Strategies for prevention of osteoporosis and hip fracture. *Br Med J*. **303**: 453–459.

Lindsay, R., MacLean, A., Kraszewski, A., Hart, D.M., Clark, A.C. and Garwood, J. (1978). Bone response to termination of oestrogen treatment. *Lancet*. **1**: 1325–1327.

Molloy, D.W., Richardson, L.D. and Grilly, R.G. (1988). The effects of a three-month exercise programme on neuropsychological function in elderly institutionalized women: a randomized controlled trial. *Age Ageing*. **17**: 303–310.

Morse, J.M., Tylko, S.J. and Dixon, H.A. (1987). Characteristics of the fall-prone patient. *Gerontologist*. **27**: 516–522.

Morton, D. (1989). Five years of fewer falls. *Am J Nurs*. **89**: 204–205.

Speechley, M. and Tinetti, M. (1991). Falls and injuries in frail and vigorous community elderly persons. *J Am Geriatr Soc*. **39**: 46–52.

Tinetti, M.E., Williams, T.F. and Mayewski, R. (1986). Fall risk index for elderly patients based on number of chronic disabilities. *Am J Med*. **80**: 429–434.

Whipple, R.H., Wolfson, L.I. and Amerman, P.M. (1987). The relationship of knee and ankle weakness to falls in Nursing Home residents: an isokinetic study. *J Am Geriatr Soc*. **35**: 13–20.

Wolf-Klein, G.P., Silverstone, F.A., Basavaraju, N., Foley, C.J., Pascaru, A. and Ma, P.-H. (1988). Prevention of falls in the elderly population. *Arch Phys Med Rehabil*. **69**: 689–691.

Wynne-Harley, D. (1991). *Living Dangerously: Risk-taking, Safety and Older People*. CPA Reports No. 16, Centre for Policy on Ageing, London.

Chapter 10 ─────────────

The future

There is no doubt that old people will continue to fall, for all the reasons outlined in the previous chapters. It is less clear, however, whether it is possible to avoid or prevent some, at least, of those falls. Despite the large amount of time and effort devoted to the study of falls, particularly over the last ten years, there are still large areas of ignorance about aspects of the problem. This is to some extent predictable, because of the enormous diversity of problems that may present as falls, but there is still scope for further work. Two things are required: better application of available information about falls and their management, and further research into causes and management of falls. Better organisation of available services could also improve management of falls and fallers. The development of orthogeriatric units is an example of what can be achieved by cooperation between different groups involved in the care of elderly fallers (Royal College of Physicians, 1989), but there is scope for further cooperation to improve services for such people.

Although individual clinicians, and sometimes departments, have more or less effective methods of dealing with elderly people who have suffered falls, what is largely lacking at present is any *systematic* assessment of fallers and their problems, in order to identify and deal with treatable causes of falling. This results in missed opportunities to prevent further falls and to improve the health and functional status of the elderly. It also results in increased pressure on health care resources. It is interesting to speculate how much money could be saved by only a small reduction in falls achieved through effective secondary prevention.

Protocols for management in various situations

There is clearly a need for well-thought-out protocols for management of elderly fallers in all the areas to which they may present, particularly where they may be dealt with by junior or non-specialist doctors. Geriatricians (at least in theory) will be aware of the multiple potential problems which may underlie the symptom, but other areas are less well prepared. Any department or facility providing for elderly people should be aware of how to assess an old person who has fallen (or should know where to direct for appropriate assessment elsewhere).

A large proportion of acute work going to orthopaedic departments now consists of elderly fallers, and there is no doubt that although many departments are aware that elderly patients with fractures have often fallen because they are ill, too many are not organised to deal optimally with ill elderly people. Their medical problems are often managed by inexperienced junior doctors with limited knowledge and skills in the care of the elderly, with sometimes inadequate back-up from their seniors. Anaesthetists often provide medical care by default to such patients, but again may not have much specialised knowledge of the elderly and their problems. Simple protocols for identifying those elderly orthopaedic patients at risk of complications of fracture or treatment and advice about management of the common problems likely to occur would improve standards of care and could speed throughput of patients. Accident Departments also often lack any well-grounded assessment procedures for falls, despite the frequency with which they are expected to manage the problem. Again, protocols to aid assessment and management of elderly fallers could improve care. There is a role for those with a special interest in the elderly, both to assist in management of their problems in Accident and Emergency Departments, and more importantly to be involved in the training of junior staff.

Risk assessment

Although some work has been carried out to allow risk of falling to be estimated in various groups of elderly people, it is preliminary and largely related to limited groups, such as those in institutional care. Further work to allow risk assessment in the elderly living at home, to aid intervention to reduce risks, is needed. The aim of such assessment would ideally be to allow risk reduction by selective interventions to improve health, mental state, environment, and so on. However, in other cases with less (or no) scope for alteration of problems, risk assessment would allow elderly people to decide what level of risk is acceptable to them to maintain their independence.

Involving patients in their own management and risk assessment

There recently has been, rightly, a change in emphasis of health care, from a paternalistic, prescriptive (and sometimes proscriptive) way of dealing with illnesses, in a very 'medical' way, to a more broadly based, multidisciplinary, holistic view of health problems. As part of this, people expect to be involved to a greater degree in decisions affecting their life and health. Because the current cohort of old people was brought up to be less questioning about their health and medical care, these new attitudes are less prevalent than in younger generations, but future cohorts will become more knowledgable and involved.

There is still a tendency for the elderly to be considered unable to make decisions about themselves and their health, with treatment decisions frequently being made largely by professionals and relatives rather than by the elderly themselves, particularly if they are frail. There needs to be empowerment of the elderly, to allow them (and therefore eventually all of us) to be involved in decisions about lifestyle and activities. This implies accepting that those decisions may not always be comfortable or without effort for those who care for the elderly, both formally and informally. The issues of balancing risk and autonomy have been discussed in Chapters 8 and 9, but once again it should be stressed that it is impossible to remove all risk of falling, and attempts to do so will almost certainly result in unacceptable restrictions of freedom and autonomy. For many elderly people, the risk of a fall resulting in a serious injury, or even death, is worth taking if independence and self-determination are maintained. That fact is often not easy for relatives and carers to live with, and the increasingly litigious atmosphere surrounding those who provide formal health and social care creates problems for those who wish to respect the freedom of people to make their own decisions, even those decisions which appear to be foolish. This becomes increasingly difficult when the old person in question is cognitively impaired, and different people have different ideas about the balance between protection and over-protection in these groups. These issues deserve greater discussion, in order to clarify acceptable codes of practice in the prevention of falls and fractures. What good is it to prevent injury if in the process quality of life is destroyed?

There needs to be an acceptance that some elderly will continue to fall despite the best efforts of health providers and carers. It follows from this that there may need to be negotiation between the patient, health professionals, carers and relatives so that all of them have a realistic appreciation about what is possible in the context of protecting the elderly from falls and their consequences, and what risks are reasonable whilst maintaining quality of life.

Nutrition and exercise

There are intriguing suggestions from previous studies about the role of nutrition and exercise in the prevention of falls and fall-related injuries. Reduced bone mass, which is a risk factor for injuries following falls, can probably be prevented by adequate dietary calcium and adequate exercise from early and middle life. There is also some evidence that exercise prevents falls by maintaining neuromuscular function and protective reflexes. It has been suggested that the epidemic of fractured neck of femur over the last few decades is a result of reduction in exercise taken by most people, not so much in the form of formal 'exercise' as the limited level of exertion required by modern life. Less developed countries have avoided the increase in incidence of 'age-related' fractures seen in North America and Europe, perhaps because of maintenance of a relatively active lifestyle (Adebajo et al., 1991).

There are worrying signs that both diet and level of exercise are becoming less healthy, and it is likely that this will add to the burden of ill-health in old age for future generations, partly manifest as falls and fractures. The most useful public health intervention to prevent the mortality and morbidity associated with falls might be to improve diet and increase opportunities for exercise for young and middle-aged people. It would, however, be difficult to prove rigorously the value of such intervention because of the complexities of studies involving behavioural change. It is likely though that the benefits of improved diet and greater exercise would have impact on many of the 'diseases of civilisation' as well as on falls and accidents.

The role of physiotherapy in the management of falls and fallers

One area which has been relatively ignored in research to date (probably because of the difficulties of designing good studies) is the role of physiotherapy and exercise in the treatment of fallers, and in the secondary prevention of falls. The physiotherapist is frequently involved in the management of elderly people with falls and balance disorders, but there is little or no information about what sorts of treatment are appropriate and how effective such treatment is. It is rightly becoming more important to demonstrate the cost-effectiveness of any intervention, and it is therefore important to know whether physiotherapy input after a fall has any effect on subsequent morbidity and independence. Consideration of psychological health would be an important part of such a study.

Dizziness and its assessment

Despite the frequency with which elderly people complain of dizziness, the symptom is at present both poorly understood, and poorly assessed and managed, both by general practitioners and hospital doctors. Otolaryngologists who have an interest in the problems of elderly people have much to offer, but only a minority of dizzy elderly are referred to ENT departments. There is no doubt that the resources of such departments would be overwhelmed if all old people complaining of dizziness were referred to them.

Education of general practitioners, in particular, about simple assessment of such patients might prevent much suffering and avoid much inappropriate prescribing. Collaboration between geriatricians and ENT surgeons might allow a district to develop specific 'dizziness' clinics, as have already been set up in some areas.

Longitudinal epidemiological studies of dizziness would add substantially to knowledge about these often vague but disabling symptoms. Cross-sectional studies have identified many of the physical, social and psychological factors which are associated with dizziness, but more information is needed about the natural history of such symptoms over time. Such information would allow intervention to be targeted. and again could prevent (or at least reduce) inappropriate drug prescription. There is also a need for research into the most effective treatments for the various types of dizziness.

Audit of management of falls and dizziness

Having thought about how to deal with an elderly person complaining of falls and/or dizziness, it is important to audit the effectiveness of assessment and management. There is a need for further work on audit of falls management, not only by specialised departments dealing with the problem, but also in primary care situations. This would help to identify which are the most cost-effective interventions and which groups of fallers are likely to benefit from them.

Outcomes

It is becoming increasingly important in all areas of health care to develop ways of measuring outcomes. In a cash-limited health care system there is inevitably going to be competition between different sectors, and demonstrating that an intervention has a beneficial outcome will be a powerful weapon in fighting for resources. Measuring outcomes for ill elderly people is not easy, and results that in younger people might be clearly unsatisfactory, such as institutionalisation or death, may in some circumstances be positive outcomes. For example, if a physically and mentally frail old person is repeatedly falling at home because of self-neglect, placement in a residential home with a high standard of care, which protects and cares for the resident whilst allowing reasonable autonomy, can result in a vast improvement in quality of life. Similarly, if falls are due to painful malignant disease, achieving a pain-free and dignified death through the provision of good quality terminal care is an appropriate outcome.

Because the problem of falls covers such a wide diversity of underlying pathological and physiological changes, determining outcomes is correspondingly difficult. This should not, however, be an excuse for failure to consider the outcome of assessments and interventions. Tools are now available to allow us to assess quality of life, for example (Fletcher et al., 1992), and such assessments could be used alongside more familiar assessments of independence and physical health. As well as death and injury following falls, such things as change in functional dependence, change in place of residence (e.g. inability to live alone or requirement for institutional care), change in mobility, and changes in psychological state should be considered as outcomes following falls and their treatment.

The topics considered in this chapter are merely a few personal thoughts about the way in which assessment and management of falls and associated problems in the elderly could be improved in the future. There are still many challenges, many questions yet to be answered, and much work yet to be done. If we are serious in our aim to 'add life to years' rather than just 'add years to life', then reducing the frequency of falls and their complications, and managing falls and their complications better when they do occur is an important part of improving quality of life for elderly people.

References

Adebajo, A.O., Cooper, C. and Evans, J.G. (1991). Fractures of the hip and distal forearm in West Africa and the United Kingdom. *Age Ageing*. **20:** 435–438.
Fletcher, A.E., Dickinson, E.J. and Philp, I. (1992). Review: audit measures: quality of life instruments for everyday use with elderly patients. *Age Ageing*. **21:** 142–150.
Royal College of Physicians (1989). *Fractured neck of femur. Prevention and management*. London, Royal College of Physicians of London.

Index